COMMUNICATION SKILLS IN
MEDICINE

COMMUNICATION SKILLS IN MEDICINE

edited by

CHARLES RK HIND BSc MD FRCP

Editor, Postgraduate Medical Journal,
London, UK; Consultant Physician,
Royal Liverpool University Hospital, and the
Cardiothoracic Centre, Liverpool, UK

BMJ
Publishing
Group

First published in 1997
by the BMJ Publishing Group, BMA House, Tavistock Square,
London WC1H 9JR

British Library Cataloguing in Publication Data

A catalogue record for this book is available from the British Library

ISBN 0-7279-1152-X

Front cover image courtesy of Ulrihe Preuss/Southampton
Community Trust

Typeset and printed by Derry, Nottingham

Contents

Contributors

Dawn L Alison
MacMillan-Robert Ogden Senior Lecturer/Honorary Consultant in Palliative Medicine and Oncology, ICRF Cancer Medicine Research Unit, St James's University Hospital, Leeds

Michael Bennet
St James's University Hospital, Leeds

Alastair W Blair
Consultant Paediatrician, Victoria Hospital, Kirkaldy, Fife

Helen L Ford
Department of Neurology, St James's University Hospital, Leeds

Charles RK Hind
Editor, the Postgraduate Medical Journal, London; Consultant Physician, Royal Liverpool University Hospital and the Cardiothoracic Centre, Liverpool

Michael H Johnson
Department of Neurology, St James's University Hospital, Leeds

Marion Miles
Consultant Paediatrician, The Medical Centre, London W9

Jonathan Marrow
Consultant in Accident and Emergency Medicine, Arrowe Park Hospital, Wirral, Merseyside

Sheila Moss
AIDS Clinical Group, Royal Liverpool University Hospital NHS Trust, Liverpool

Barbara M Phillips
Consultant in Paediatric Emergency Medicine, Alder Hey Children's Hospital, Liverpool

Steven Ryan
Senior Lecturer in Neonatal and Paediatric Medicine, Institute of Child Health, Alder Hey Children's Hospital, Liverpool

Simon J Sherwood
Department of Psychology, University of Edinburgh, Edinburgh

Sam Smith
Honorary Lecturer, Department of Primary Care, Whelan Building, Liverpool

Roger D Start
Department of Pathology, Chesterfield Hospital, Chesterfield

Christopher R Steer
Consultant Paediatrician, Victoria Hospital, Kirkaldy, Fife

Kevin Stewart
Consultant Physician, Medicine and Elderly Care, Royal Hampshire County Hospital, Winchester, Hampshire

Anthony K Webb
Consultant Chest Physician, Bradbury Cystic Fibrosis Unit, Wythenshawe Hospital, Manchester

Olwen E Williams
Department of Genitourinary Medicine, Wrexham Maelor Hospital NHS Trust, Wrexham, Clwyd

Introduction

CHARLES RK HIND

Communication is of central importance in health care. It is necessary for the science of medicine, through the elucidation of symptoms and signs. It also underpins the art of medicine through its concern with both the uniqueness of the individual patient, and the impact of the disease or disorder on that patient (box 1). Through this latter quality, it is also the start of the therapeutic process, or in other situations the start of the mourning process.

Box 1—The ideal doctor

"Generosity he has, such as is possible to those who practise an art, never to those who drive a trade; discretion, tested by a hundred secrets; tact, tried in a thousand embarassments; and what are more important, Hearaclean cheerfulness and courage. So it is he brings an air and cheer into the sickroom, and often enough, though not so often as he wishes, brings healing".

RL Stevenson (1850-1894)

For many decades, the acquisition of the necessary skills to communicate bad news to patients or relatives has come by "osmosis" or by "experience". The latter was defined by Oscar Wilde as "the name every one gives to their mistakes". More recently the importance of the formal teaching of such skills has been recognised, not only at undergraduate level, but also at junior and senior postgraduate level. The 13 chapters in this book provide a clear understanding of how to approach the commonest clinical situations in which such communication skills are paramount. Each provides the reader with a detailed "How to" approach to that clinical situation, together with a clear reminder of possible pitfalls.

Through each chapter run nine general themes, which for the basic framework for ensuring that these communication skills are practised well in every clinical situation (box 2).

Box 2—Guidelines to good communication skills in medicine

- time
- preparation
- ability to be honest and compassionate
- ability to express feeling
- ability to listen
- ability to explain
- ability to understand
- ability to care
- consistency

Time

Firstly, time to learn the necessary skills. Before breaking bad news to a patient or relative, the doctor must have acquired the necessary skills. This takes time, and if that doctor feels unready, then the help of a more senior doctor must be requested.

Secondly, time to talk to the patient or relative, and to address their various concerns. For the busy clinician, breaking bad news is just one of numerous tasks that have to be squeezed into the day. In contrast, for the patient or family in crisis, that interaction with the doctor is likely to be a unique, never-forgotten event. Somehow the busy clinician must act like a true professional, and appear to have all the time in the world to undertake the task in hand.

Thirdly, time for the patient or relative to realise the gravity or seriousness of the situation. And time, according to the particular clinical setting, for the patient or relative to be involved in any decision-making (eg, to have surgery or chemotherapy for their cancer). If necessary, a second interview should be planned for the next day or week, to give the patient or relative time to discuss the options with other relatives, friends or health care professionals. The pace of the interview should be dictated by the patient or relative, and not by the doctor.

Preparation

Firstly, it is vital that the doctor has spent as long as is necessary becoming familiar with all of the aspects of the case, with the assistance of other appropriate health care workers.

Secondly, the interview should take place in a private and quiet area. The emphasis should be on good manners, such as standing when the patient or relative enters the room, introducing yourself to all present ("Good morning, Mrs Smith. My name is Dr Hind, and I am a chest consultant"), finding out exactly who is present at the interview and their relation to the patient in question, and shaking each by the hand.

Thirdly, preparing the ground by finding out from the patient or relative either what other doctors or health care workers have already said to them, or what their immediate concerns are (or both).

Ability to be honest and compassionate

Doctors need the ability to give the bad news gently and honestly, but with the compassion of a fellow human being (eg, "I'm sorry to say this, but yes, the diagnosis is one of cancer"). Honesty may also be required by the more junior doctor who is dealing with a problem at a time when more senior medical help is not available (eg, talking to relatives in the middle of the night, following an unexpected death). A polite but honest admission that the doctor is not in a position to answer all the relatives questions at that time is the best approach, provided that doctor ensures a more senior doctor is available as soon as is possible the next working day to address any unanswered questions.

Ability to express feelings

Though the reaction of the patient or relative to the bad news will vary, certain reactions are commoner than others (see chapter 1). Familiarity with the commoner reactions beforehand will allow the doctor to be prepared as to how to respond.

Ability to listen

The doctor must avoid any natural inclination to dominate the conversation. Having started the ball rolling with an honest but direct appraisal of the facts (see above), the doctor must then allow the pace and the direction of the subsequent discussion to be determined by the patient or relative. A considerable amount of medical knowledge may be needed at this stage by the doctor, to answer the points raised by the patient or relatives (eg, see chapter 4).

Ability to explain

All the concerns raised must be addressed by the doctor with honesty, and in a way understandable to someone who may not have had the same educational advantages as the doctor (box 3). If the doctor cannot answer all of the questions raised, this must be honestly and openly acknowledged, and arrangements made for the patient or relative to see someone who can address any outstanding issues.

Box 1—Being a good listener

"Doctors must be good listeners...—and they must be able to provide advice and explanations that are comprehensible".

General Medical Council, London, UK, 1995

Ability to understand

In these situations, the doctor should not be afraid to reply to a question from the patient or relative, by asking a further question. This may allow the doctor to discover why the question was asked in the first place. For example, the cancer patient who asks about prognosis may only be asking this question to discover whether he will still be in a position to walk his daughter down the aisle in three months time. Only be determining the real reason behind the question, will the doctor be able to address the issue to the full satisfaction of the patient.

Ability to care

It is often the period after the doctor has left that is the more difficult time for the patient or relative whose world has just been turned upside down. The caring doctor will ensure that the patient or relative has not been left in a void, by ensuring that a health care worker is present, close by, or at the end of the telephone, to help them come to terms with the situation, and perhaps reinforce or clarify what has been said.

Consistency

Consistency amongst the various health care workers in terms of the information given to a patient or relative is vital. The importance of making a clear written record of every interview with the patient or a relative cannot be overemphasised. The doctor should also make certain that all the other health care workers involved (eg, family doctor, cancer nurse specialist) are fully appraised of what the patient or relative has been told.

I hope that the following thirteen chapters provide the necessary insight to the doctor or trainee, which, as Oliver Wendell Holmes once said, is sometimes worth a lifetime's experience.

Charles RK Hind

1 Talking to the parents of a baby with perinatal brain insults

STEVEN RYAN

What brain insults occur?

In most children who develop a neurological impairment in childhood, there is no acute perinatal illness. Although Little assumed that most cerebral palsy was due to birth asphyxia,[1] we now know that probably less than 10% of cases result from such asphyxia. However, in any reasonably sized maternity unit, there will be several babies born each year with acute disorders of the brain who are at risk of long-term impairment.

The commonest disorders encountered are hypoxic-ischaemic encephalopathy, most commonly seen in full term neonates, and

---

Box 1.1 Acquired conditions causing perinatal brain injury

- intrapartum asphyxia, eg, placental abruption, ruptured uterus, cord prolapse
- preterm infants: intraventricular haemorrhage, periventricular leukomalacia
- kernicterus
- meningitis
- intracerebral haemorrhage: vascular malformation, coagulopathy
- trauma
- encephalitis, eg, cytomegalovirus

1

intraventricular haemorrhage and periventricular leucomalacia in preterm neonates. Because these conditions are relatively common, relatively large series of cases have been reported, establishing the relationship between the severity of the initial illness and long-term outcome. Using this information it becomes possible to give the parents some idea of their child's likely outcome. Other rarer causes of brain insult in the perinatal period are kernicterus (hyperbilirubinaemic encephalopathy) and meningitis (box 1).

Hypoxic-ischaemic encephalopathy

Clinically, hypoxic-ischaemic encephalopathy (figure 1.1) has been divided into three grades and this grading system is now widely used. Levene *et al*[2] showed that neonates with mild encephalopathy (no seizures) had virtually no risk of long-term disability, those with moderate encephalopathy had a risk of about 25% of dying or having a severe disability and those with severe encephalopathy had a risk between 50% and 100% of a similar outcome. Other features which are associated with high risk of adverse outcome are delayed onset of spontaneous respiration beyond 20 minutes, a delay in feeding beyond the age of a week and a persisting abnormal neurological status in the newborn period. In infants suffering a cardiac arrest at birth, all survivors not breathing spontaneously at 30 minutes developed spastic quadriplegia.[3] In another study 75% of infants not breathing spontaneously by 20 minutes after birth either died or had severe neurological impairment.[4]

Persisting hypotonia or hypotonia rapidly evolving to extensor hypertonia is associated with a high incidence (>75%) of either death or handicap.[2] In many infants, however, particularly in the group with moderate encephalopathy, there is a "honeymoon" period of several months when the infant appears to have no or little neurological abnormality. In this situation it is wise to be cautious. In most infants by one year of age any abnormality, most usually cerebral palsy, will reveal itself. In general, the earlier the abnormality is detected, the more severe the resulting impairment.

Intraventricular haemorrhage

Intraventricular haemorrhage arises in preterm neonates from the germinal matrix lying bilaterally in the floor of the body of the

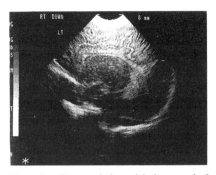

Figure 1.1 Parasaggital cranial ultrasound of fullterm neonate with enhanced gyral pattern and slit-like lateral ventricle, due to cerebral oedema

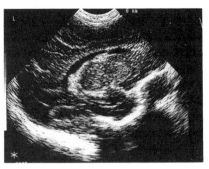

Figure 1.2 Left sided parasaggital cranial ultrasound scan of preterm infant showing sub-ependymal haemorrhage as echodensity on floor of body of lateral ventricle

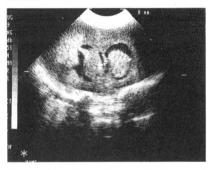

Figure 1.3 Coronal cranial ultrasound through anterior fossa of preterm neonate showing bilateral echodense clots within dilated anterior horns of both lateral ventricles. On one side venous infarction has led to an echodensity within the parenchyma

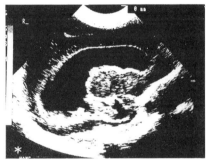

Figure 1.4 Parasaggital cranial ultrasound scan in preterm neonate showing post-haemorrhagic ventricular dilatation

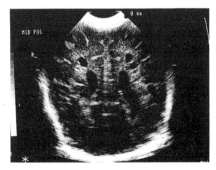

Figure 1.5 Posterior coronal cranial ultrasound scan in preterm neonate showing bilateral occipital cystic leukomalacia. This appearance is strongly correlated with severe multiple neurological disability

3

lateral ventricle next to the head of the caudate nucleus. Haemorrhage may be confined to the matrix (Grade I; figure 1.2), in which case impairment is unlikely. If the haemorrhage ruptures into the ventricle itself (Grade II; figure 1.3), this may cause obstruction to flow of cerebrospinal fluid—post haemorrhagic hydrocephalus (figure 1.4), or local parenchymal infarction (figure 1.3). In either of these situations, there is a high risk of long-term impairment, cerebral palsy being common.[5] If an infant requires treatment for post-haemorrhagic ventricular dilatation in the newborn period, there is a 90% risk of neuromotor impairment which results in 76% of survivors having a marked disability[5]. Other impairments include deficits in vision, hearing, and intellect. Bilateral lesions have a greater association with severe impairments. All haemorrhagic lesions are easily identified by cranial ultrasound in the neonatal period.[6]

Ischaemic lesions in preterm infants occur in the periventricular area, which is the vascular watershed at low gestations. Lesions occur in up to 5% of preterm neonates up to 32 weeks gestation. Significant lesions are usually bilateral and result in "punched-out" cystic lesions seen on cranial ultrasound[6] (figure 1.5) above and lateral to the ventricles. Cerebral palsy is frequently seen, since the internal capsules pass through this area. Diplegia is more commonly seen than quadriplegia.[7]

Withdrawing care?

It is obviously possible to identify some infants in the first days who are at very high risk of death or severe handicap. If such infants are receiving intensive care, it may be appropriate to consider withdrawing it. This situation will not be discussed further in this article except to say that the final decision must be taken by the senior clinician in charge of the patient's care. The situation must be explained to the parents and they must understand and accept the decision before it is enacted. However, the parents must not feel that they were responsible for making the choice. It is not within the scope of this chapter to discuss the ethics underlying such a decision.

What do parents want to know?

Parents want to know what has happened, why it has happened and what it means for the future of their child? In explaining what has happened, simple terms such as brain damage are acceptable, particularly if the parents understand and use the term. There is always the temptation for doctors to give a large amount of technical medical detail, quite often at a level we would not expect medical students to comprehend fully! If there are any scan images, show them to the infant's parents, since this helps get your message over. If possible, have a normal scan available for comparison. Scan images are most helpful for haemorrhagic lesions in preterm neonates, as ultrasound images in babies with even severe encephalopathy can be normal or exhibit subtle changes (figure 1.1).

An explanation of the reasons for their child's predicament will be high on the parents' agenda. They will need to know if anything could have been done differently which would have prevented the situation. Brain lesions in preterm infants arise as a consequence of prematurity. There is little evidence to suggest that avoidable obstetric factors have any influence on the incidence of these problems.

The parents of an infant who appears to have suffered intra-partum birth asphyxia, may be very concerned to find out if any such factors existed. It is said that inadequacy in dealing with such questions and failure to apologise if an inadequacy has occurred are the root of much litigation. So the issue must be addressed. Ideally the obstetrician in charge of the mother's care should address such issues as soon as possible, answering all of the parents' questions. He or she should be aware of what the parents have been told by the paediatrician.

Paediatricians should be aware, however, that some babies who appear asphyxiated are not. Babies may have developed or acquired an abnormality of the central nervous system before labour. Such babies can present with all the classical features of intra-partum asphyxia because their ability to react to the stressful event of labour is impaired. Abnormal cardiotocograms, meconium-stained liquor, depressed Apgar score and neonatal encephalopathy have all been described in such infants.[8,9] Of course, their abnormal central nervous system results in future neurological impairment. Hence the term birth asphyxia should be used with caution. In the first instance, a purely descriptive "label" of features present should be attached. If necessary, this concept should be explained to the parents.

Having established that a disorder has arisen, the parents will

5

want to know what this means for the future of their child. They would like an accurate picture but unfortunately this is not always possible. For instance in a fullterm neonate who has suffered moderately severe hypoxic–ischaemic encephalopathy, the average risk of severe problems is 25%. The problem is that it is impossible to know for the individual child, whether he or she is in that 25% or the other 75%. Rather than hazarding a guess, it is important to explain this uncertainty. If you can show that you are "confident" about this uncertainty and you are familiar with up-to-date opinion, you can still develop a trusting relationship with the parents. It is all right to say "I do not know".

One useful way of getting the message over is by referring to a range of potential disabilities; an equivalent, say, to a confidence interval between the 5th and 95th centile. Here you can set out for the parents the nature of the best and worst outcomes they could expect. For instance the child who has suffered moderately severe hypoxic–ischaemic encephalopathy has one goal post which is normality and another which represents spastic quadriplegia and severe compromise of future lifestyle. It is wise to avoid, at this stage of uncertainty, specific statements about likely function. If asked "Will she walk?" in the above scenario, you can return to the range of disabilities you have predicted as potential outcomes. There is evidence that even accurate statements, if given in a pessimistic context, give rise to anger, which can be lifelong, eg, "your child will never read or write".[10] Here the idea of a range is useful as it gives the parents some target to aim for and allows some optimism.

The lack of specificity should be accompanied by some idea of when you are likely to be more certain and what follow-up you intend. By the age of nine months to a year, most cerebral palsy will have revealed itself.

Breaking the news

In many ways delivering news of a likely or impending handicap is like telling relatives that a family member has died. The parents will have had some image of how their normal child was going to live. This loss of that potential provokes a grief reaction which can be as intense as that seen in a bereavement. Similar skills, facilities, and resources to those needed when imparting the news of a death are required. The parents' experience at the initial informing interview can play an important role in the family's perception of the child and their long-term adjustment to the child's disability.[11] Consequently, it is not only important what is communicated, but how it is communicated.

If possible, parents should be told together. They should be told as soon as a likely problem is identified, sympathetically and

---

Box 1.2 What parents want of their doctor

- familiar to parent
- already knows child
- appears comfortable
- equal not superior
- supportive

Box 1.3 What information parents want

- co-ordinated
- clear
- includes positive characteristics
- addresses future questions
- resources available
- share diagnostic features (scans, etc)

Box 1.4 How parents want to be told

Delivery

- direct
- caring, compassionate
- information personalised
- gradual–paced, not hurried

Situation

- private and quiet
- face to face (not telephone)
- parents together, with supporters
- baby present
- parents have already spent time with baby

without jargon.[10] Parents appreciate being told directly in a clear straightforward way but including positive images of their child (boxes 1.2-1.4).[10]

Understand nature of parental reaction

The parents' reaction can be very intense and can include inappropriate feelings of anxiety, guilt or blame. Firstly, the parents should be told that these reactions are normal human emotional reactions to such a situation. Secondly, it is necessary to allay these inappropriate feelings. This process may have to be repeated several times. By knowing the nature of the reaction, the medical team can be prepared and know that it is not their actions in breaking the news which have been the cause of such feelings. It will also make them aware that the parents may feel anger and blame and direct it at their child's carers. In some senses an obvious emotional reaction is a sign that the message has got across.

Setting up the interview

Having the infant's nurse with you when you break the news has several advantages. Firstly, support for yourself and secondly in ensuring a consistent message to the parents. It is helpful to brief the nurse prior to the interview to explain the main points you wish to raise. He or she may also be able to retain some of the parents' questions which they overlook. The nurse will also be able to reiterate the main messages until the next interview and log any further questions the parents may have. The nurse can also translate any medical jargon inadvertently used. A junior medical colleague can also perform many of the same roles and will also obtain useful training. By asking the nurse or medical colleague about what they thought you did well and what they would have done differently, the interviewer can gain valuable insight into his or her own technique. In this situation it is important to avoid negative feedback, as this can itself be distressing in such circumstances.

Following the interview a comprehensive medical note should be written. This serves as an important communication for other health care workers and helps to ensure a consistent message. The nurse should also record his or her perceptions in the nursing cardex.

Parents appreciate privacy and time when being given bad news, and up to 45 minutes should be allowed for the first session. A frequent reaction to the delivery of the news is stunned silence, or crying. One's natural instinct at this point is to try and break the silence or perhaps leave. Another approach is to remain silent and wait for the parents to ask you the next question. This rarely takes more than one or two minutes. At this time the parents will hardly seem to notice your presence and in hindsight they frequently comment that knowing the doctor was still available was helpful. Having the baby present with you at the time is helpful, but this may not be possible if the baby is unwell and on a busy special care unit.

The first interview should be the start of a number of interviews, which are arranged at the time of the first interview. These secondary interviews should have the format of the first, but concentrate even more on answering the parents' questions and checking they have understood the main concepts. Occasionally, due to unforseen circumstances, another doctor may be asked to undertake an interview, possibly requested at short notice by the parents. In this situation a review of the nursing and medical notes and open questions to the parents about their current understanding will usually allow a successful interview.

Parents appreciate a doctor who is empathic, who listens and who seems to understand them.[10] This appreciation can be fostered by such simple methods as furniture placement and posture, and knowledge of other basic communication skills.[11] Not the cold distant upright figure the other side of a desk, but the doctor sitting with the parents, sitting forward attentively. There is some question about the degree of physical contact. A hug? A handshake? A hand on the shoulder? There is no set way. Do what you feel comfortable with.

At some point during the interviews, tell the parents that you do not mind them bringing written questions, since it will aid their memory of and understanding of any points which you make.

Cerebral palsy

The most frequent adverse outcome in survivors of neonatal brain disorders is cerebral palsy. Since the definition of the condition continues to be debated, great care is required when informing the parents about the condition. The parents may have their own idea about what constitutes cerebral palsy, so before the interviewer describes the condition, the parents should be asked what they understand by the term. If they have a fair idea, this will aid communication. If their knowledge is false or unrealistic, finding out at this stage will enable the interviewer to correct misapprehensions. This will remove significant barriers to communication.

The most commonly accepted definitions of cerebral palsy suggest a brain disorder arising in the perinatal period which damages the motor pathways. This results in abnormalities of tone (and hence posture) and motor control. Explaining that the medical term "spastic" refers to this increased tone is helpful. Once the lesion is established it is non-progressive, another important concept. Depending on the nature of brain insult, it may be possible to outline the most frequent pattern of cerebral palsy seen with it. Kernicterus and very late perinatal acute asphyxia for instance are both associated with the development of dyskinetic athetoid cerebral palsy.[12]

Written information at this point can be helpful in getting the message across. Some texts are written for parents rather than professionals and can be helpful in allowing the parents to formulate more specific questions.[13] An outline of any early interventions (such as physiotherapy), their rationale and benefit will be a positive message for the parents.[14]

Planning for the future

In addition to breaking the bad news, it is important to give some positive message. One concept worth introducing is the plastic nature of the neonatal brain which allows occasional remarkable degrees of functionality to return. The parents' role in aiding this process should be stressed, giving them a positive role as soon as possible. The concept of their child's potential is one that parents accept and grasp readily. Remembering the concept of the range of potential outcomes above, it can be expressed in terms of the number of agencies and people who will help their child over the first few years. Lack of awareness of speciality referrals and community services is perceived badly.[10]

Some services, such as those provided by the family doctor and health visitor, they will already be familiar with. There are also likely to be local or national organisations who have a great deal to

---

Box 1.5 Enhancing communication

● listen
● check parents' understanding at each interview
● meet parents several times
● have a nurse present
● ask parents to write down their questions
● use any scans or images or demonstrate physical signs to the parents

---

offer these families, including counselling as well as practical help. SCOPE, the British organisation dedicated to helping people with cerebral palsy, is one example. The hospital social worker will have a list of contacts for such organisations.

Learning how to do it

How can you learn or improve the skills needed for this task? The first step is to sit in during a consultation in which bad news is being given. This, as described above, has the potential for training for both the exponent and the observer. A well-defined positive-feedback "system" is available to ensure that the exponent does not feel threatened. Role play, though seemingly disliked by many, can in the right format be a very effective tool for improving communication skills and raising issues. Texts are also available giving an overview of communication between health professionals and their patients, and used with practical or role-playing experience can help with identifying specific areas for attention and improvement.[11]

In summary the basic communication skills needed in this situation are no different from those used generally. An understanding of parental reaction to the breaking of bad news is helpful. Boxes 1.2-1.5 adapted from Krahn *et al*,[10] give a list of parental concerns which informers should attempt to address.

---

1   Little WJ. On the influence of abnormal parturition, difficult labours, premature birth, and asphyxia neonatorum, on the mental and physical condition of the child, especially in relation to deformities. *Trans Obstet Soc London* 1862;3:293-344.

2   Levene MI. The asphyxiated newborn infant. In: Levene MI, Bennett MJ, Punt J, eds. *Fetal and neonatal neurology and neurosurgery*, 1st edn. Edinburgh: Churchill Livingstone, 1988; pp 370-82.

3   Steiner H, Neligan G. Perinatal cardiac arrest: quality of survivors. *Arch Dis Child* 1975;**50**:596-702.

4   Ergander U, Eriksson M, Zetterstrom R. Severe neonatal asphyxia: incidence and prediction of outcome in the Stockholm area. *Acta Paeditr Scand* 1983;**72**:321-5.

5   Ventriculomegaly Trial Group. Randomised trial of early tapping in neonatal posthaemorrhagic ventricular dilatation: results at 30 months. *Arch Dis Child* 1994;**70**:141-6.

6   Ryan SW. Cranial ultrasound in the newborn. In: Carty H, Shaw D, Brunelle F, Kendall B, eds. *Imaging children*. 1st edn, Vol 2. Edinburgh: Churchill Livingstone, 1994; pp 1426-39.

7   De Vries LS, Larroche JC, Levene MI. Cerebral ischaemic lesions. In: Levene MI, Bennett MJ, Punt J, eds. *Fetal and neonatal neurology and neurosurgery*, 1st edn. Edinburgh: Churchill Livingston, 1988; pp 326-38.

8   Gaffney G, Flavell V, Johnson A, Squier M, Sellers S. Cerebral palsy and neonatal encephalopathy. *Arch Dis Child* 1994;**70**:F195-200.

9   Naeye RL, Peters EC, Bartholomew M, Landis R. Origins of cerebral palsy. *Am J Dis Child* 1989;**143**:1154-61.

10   Krahn GL, Hallum A, Kime C. Are there good ways to give 'bad news'. *Paediatrics* 1993;**91**:578-82.

11   Smith VM, Bass TA, eds. *Communication for health professionals*, 1st edn. Philadelphia: JB Lipincott Company, 1979.

12   Rosenbloom L. Dyskinetic cerebral palsy and birth asphyxia. *Dev Med Child Neurol* 1994;**36**:285-9.

13   Finnie NR, ed. *Handling the young cerebral palsied child at home*, 2nd edn. London: William Heinemann Medical, 1981.

14   Scrutton D, ed. *Management of the motor disorders of children with cerebral palsy*, 1st edn. London: Spastics International Medical Publications, 1984.

2 Telling parents their child has severe congenital anomalies

STEVEN RYAN

Background

The birth of babies with major congenital anomalies is becoming less common in the UK. The reduction in incidence is due to the identification of malformed fetuses by medical screening in early pregnancy and their subsequent termination, but in some conditions, such as spina bifida, there has been a fall in the conception of affected fetuses. Many expectant parents feel that there is no chance of their baby having a malformation and many will not have considered such an outcome.

There has been a major change in attitude over life-saving treatment for children with life-threatening malformations. For instance, infants with Down's syndrome are now more likely to be offered corrective surgery for atrioventricular septal defects and duodenal atresia.[1]

When are abnormalities detected?

Some parents will have been made aware that their unborn child has a major abnormality, but they may have chosen to continue with the pregnancy despite this. The involvement of a paediatrician before birth allows the condition and its natural history to be better defined, parents' questions answered and plans made for the delivery and postnatal care. The parents can visit the neonatal unit. A description of the most likely postnatal course will be helpful for the parents and, if surgery is contemplated, so will an interview with the surgeon. Videotapes of interviews with parents of children

13

with malformations have been prepared as an aid to antenatal counselling.[2] Parents shown the film described it as useful and accurate; more so than genetic health visitors who also saw it. The authors used this discrepancy to call for a more balanced and non-directive approach from professionals involved in antenatal counselling.

When a major malformation is identified at birth, all efforts should be made to keep the baby with his or her mother. There is a natural reaction, born of apprehension, to remove the child for assessment to another room or to the special care baby unit. This interferes with the natural bonding process with the mother. For example, a child who is immediately put to the breast has an increased chance of successful breast feeding. It is unnecessary for every baby with a malformation to be removed to the special care baby unit, individual assessment being required. The chances of parental rejection are increased if the mother and baby are separated.[3] Babies with cleft palate or Down's syndrome can frequently be nursed on the postnatal ward with their mothers.

When first talking to the parents, the baby should be present, firstly allowing important physical signs to be shown and secondly to remove the element of the unknown.[4] The parents' imagination may suggest a more "horrifying" malformation than actually exists. When a child has been born with a cleft lip or other external abnormality, in addition to demonstrating the physical features, showing the parents pictures of other babies before and after surgery can be very reassuring. If possible a selection of pictures of varying severity of lesions should be available.

A baby with an important malformation may appear normal to his or her parents. This may be the case in the parents of a child with Down's syndrome. Frequently however, such parents later

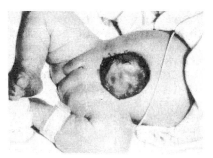

Figure 2.1 Exomphalos

admit to noticing that their child is different, but have said nothing because it has not been confirmed by the birth attendants. In other situations, the staff's unusual reaction to the delivery alerts the mother to some problem.[5] Occasionally malformations which look similar can have very different prognoses. Exomphalos (figure 2.1), for example, is associated with a number of other potentially serious malformations, whereas gastroschisis is not.

When to interview the parents

If a malformation is evident or strongly suspected, the parents should be told as soon as possible. Where they express a preference, most parents say they wish to know as soon as the staff suspected a problem.[4-6] It is sometimes suggested that confirmatory diagnostic tests should be completed prior to talking to the parents. In fact *informed* consent is required to obtain samples for diagnostic tests. For example, in a baby with suspected Down's syndrome the clinical diagnosis is usually certain. The karyotype is analysed for conformation of the diagnosis and also to detect the small number of cases which are inherited by chromosomal translocation.

Previously, it was suggested that parents should be told as soon as a definitive rather than suspected diagnosis was made, and, if there were any uncertainty, to await confirmation or the parents' first approach.[3] Nowadays the norm is to keep the parents informed, even in the presence of uncertainty.

The interview

Perhaps as many as 50% of mothers are dissatisfied with the way a disability is disclosed or discussed with them,[7] a finding not dependent on the profession of the teller. The earliest opportunity should be taken, when both parents are present and when a senior clinician is available, to conduct an interview. If one of the parents or such a clinician is unavailable, the pros and cons of breaking the news to the mother alone by a more junior doctor have to be weighed up. In any event, where a malformation is obvious, this should be discussed immediately. When confirmatory tests are required parental consent is required, so the reasons for the test must be explained to the parents.

The most effective form of communication with parents, as in

Box 2.1 Common communication problems of doctors

- premature interruption of patient
- lack of insight of what's important to the patient
- lack of explanation
- not seeking feedback or checking patient's or carers' understanding
- unclear or complicated information
- use of jargon

---

all situations,[8] involves listening and answering questions. The least effective form of communication is to bombard the parents with a mass of medical facts. If one stops to consider, it is apparent that one is trying to get parents to understand concepts we only expect medical students to grasp after intensive study. In the uncomfortable situation of breaking "bad" news, it is easy for the health professional to lapse into a lecture. This often helps us cope with the situation and fills awkward silences. But silences are not awkward; they are signs of effective communication and allow time for thought. They allow time for questions. Common problems with doctor–patient communication are shown in box 2.1.[8] Some solutions are shown in box 2.2. These are general principles of communication, but apply equally to this situation.

Box 2.2 Features of good communication

Elicit all main concerns from patient/parent by:

- active listening
- empathy
- summarise
- use of open-ended questions
- clear explanations
- checking understanding, clarify when required

One way to deliver such news is to make a first statement which is bold and simple: "I think that your baby has Down's syndrome", "Your child has a serious heart disorder". Parents appreciate a direct approach—"not beating around the bush".[4,5] At that point remain silent. The parents may immediately react in an emotional manner or may simply ask you "What is Down's syndrome?". By allowing the parents to "drive" the interview you can go at their pace and at their level of understanding. Try and avoid long lists of medical words. Avoid medical jargon. At this early stage, you are just trying to communicate the main points. For instance with Down's syndrome you should be allowing the parents to understand that their child is likely to have learning difficulties and may have associated malformations. You do not need to bog them down in minutiae such as the requirement for thyroid function screening in later life. It is also important that the parents continue to perceive themselves as the main decision makers in matters concerning their child. It is easy to overlook this role in complex situations.[5] Choices should be made by parents, based on clear understanding of medical issues.

The direct approach also avoids the trap of asking the parents to make the diagnosis by revealing physical signs to them. Further information on parents' needs during these early interviews is contained within another article in this series.[9]

Parents are unhappy if they are told abruptly and without apparent sympathy or concern, cannot understand what has been said or if they feel they have been misled or fobbed off.[5] Features of the disclosure which make parents more satisfied are shown in box 2.3.[7] The key elements which parents rated the most highly were the professional's manner, adequate information, and the opportunity to ask questions.

Box 2.3 What makes parents more satisfied with disclosure?

- opportunities to ask questions
- opportunity to contact teller again
- information easily understandable, easy to remember, and adequate quantity
- informant sympathetic, understanding, a good communicator, direct, approachable and open

---

A single interview is unlikely to be adequate, so that at the end of the first, follow-up interviews should be arranged. On subsequent occasions the parents should be encouraged to bring a list of written questions with them, since it is easy to forget important points when others are being discussed at length. The primary nurse or midwife for the parents and child should also be present. At the start of second and subsequent interviews it is useful to ask the parents to recall what they already understand. This is especially useful if the earlier interview, was conducted by a colleague.

Box 2.4 A "model service" for breaking the news[5]

- interview by consultant with specialist health visitor
- as soon as possible—except if poor maternal health
- parents together
- private room, no disturbance
- infant present in room unless ill
- as much time as necessary for questions
- balanced viewpoint, not exhaustive list of potential problems
- specialist health visitor available at parents request
- privacy continues after interview for parents
- follow-up interview within 24 hours

Cunningham and colleagues set up a "model service" to inform parents that their newborn child had Down's syndrome (box 2.4). This model service, significantly improved the satisfaction of parents with disclosure.[5] The *Right From The Start* strategy working group (see appendix for address) has also produced a template of skills and attitudes which provide a philosophical and practical guide to disclosure.

Parents feel happier if they are presented with a positive image of their child.[4,5] This is helped if the child is with them when they are interviewed. By not initiating the interview with the phrase such as "I have some bad news for you", a more positive outlook can be initiated. Other positive messages include the potential which all children have, and the positive efforts which health and other services will undertake to secure the child's maximum potential, emphasising the value which we place on the child's future. Even accurate information, delivered in an unduly pessimistic way may elicit anger in parents.[4] Early support, which allows parents to feel they can help their child to develop towards

18

their full potential from an early stage, is crucial.[10]

Understanding the emotional impact of the situation upon the parents and understanding that failure to produce a good outcome

---

Box 2.5 Typical emotional reaction in new parents of a child with a malformation[10]

- *biological*
  protection of the helpless
  revulsion at abnormality
- *inadequacy*
  of reproduction
  of rearing
- *bereavement*
  loss of normal child expected
  anger, grief and adjustment
- feelings of shock, guilt, embarrassment and helplessness

---

occurs despite our best efforts, augments the physician's ability to communicate. It also removes from the physician the responsibility for the emotional suffering which is itself inevitable and natural.[4,11] The nature of the parental emotional response has been well described and is summarised in box 2.5.[10] Box 2.6 lists ways in which this emotional response may manifest. The seeking of a second or further opinion by the parents is not a sign of failure on the part of the doctor.[10]

Box 2.6 Manifestations of the emotional reaction in parents

- *depression*
  lack of confidence
  inconsistent child care
- *disbelief*
  succession of medical opinions
  seeking good news
- *aggression*
  blame
- *rejection*
  cold, calculated
  dutiful or theatrical care without warmth
- withdrawal from social contacts

The parents will almost certainly want to ask why their child has the problem and, if it is only discovered postnatally, why the panoply of modern antenatal care did not detect it. Such a question could be directed to the obstetricians or midwives involved in antenatal care.

Commonly the parents, and especially the mother, may feel personally responsible for their child's malformation. In virtually all circumstances this feeling is unreasonable and inappropriate. Since most parents experience this feeling at some time, it is worth seeking out with a direct question if it has not been previously mentioned, so that guilt may be allayed.

Other information sources including referral

What caused the malformation? Will it happen in future pregnancies? The initiating event in most malformations is still unknown, but is being increasingly described for a variety of malformations. The field of clinical and molecular genetics is moving so rapidly, that it is wise to seek the opinion of a clinical geneticist, so that the very latest information is available for the parents.

If the parents are contemplating future pregnancies and the risk of a further malformed child is increased, they will wish to know what specialised antenatal care will be available, particularly with respect to antenatal diagnosis. The parents should be referred to a consultant obstetrician with special experience in fetal medicine. This allows the couple to contemplate a further pregnancy with reassurance.

If treatment, including surgery, is contemplated, this will need to be discussed. In the acquisition of informed consent, the nature of the problem, its natural history and the risks and benefits of the proposed intervention will need to be covered. If time permits, a number of separate interviews will ensure good communication and fully informed consent. Sometimes urgent life-saving treatment is required and a single interview must suffice. Written information is very useful in such circumstances. Parent information documents can be produced for the more commonly encountered conditions, detailing the points above. The advent of good quality printers and readily available personal computers allows such documents to be produced when needed rather than gathering dust and getting lost. Videos are particularly well understood by parents.

Other sources of information

There are a number of other sources of information available. Medical texts may give useful information to the parents, but do require vetting. Be particularly careful with older textbooks, which contain inaccurate information, particularly regarding prognosis.[2] Their views are frequently based on selective groups of patients, seen before the advent of modern screening methods. The best information is usually found in recent state-of-the-art reviews in medical journals. You should consider reviewing the article with the parents to answer their questions and to decipher the medical language for them. Most parents appreciate having the information, and it reveals your willingness to share fully your information. Such documents may contain references to difficult areas, such as the risk of leukaemia in Down's syndrome. The doctor needs to be aware of the presence of such information and be prepared to deal with questions on it.

Some information sources are specifically designed for parents and carers. They are frequently produced by organisations and charities formed to represent the interests of children and their carers. SOFT UK (Support Organisation for Trisomy 13/18 and related disorders) is an example (see appendix). The doctor has usually not been in the situation of having a child with the malformation, and is therefore unlikely to guess all the parents concerns and questions. Other parents, however, are likely to have many common experiences and questions and these organisations draw on this valuable resource when compiling information documents. Local branches of such organisations may be able to arrange for the parents to meet other parents who have a child with the malformation. They may also be able to offer practical help. MENCAP (Royal Society for Mentally Handicapped Children and Adults) is a UK organisation which provides nursery placement for such infants (see appendix).

Most of these organisations provide introductory pamphlets, useful for both parents and professionals alike (figures 2.2 and 2.3 and see appendix). It is worthwhile obtaining as many as these pamphlets as possible, for future use.

Many of these organisations are large, multinational and

21

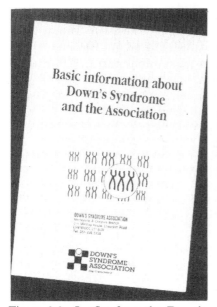

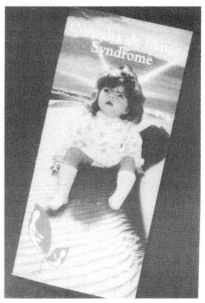

Figure 2.2 Leaflet from the Down's Syndrome Association

Figure 2.3 Leaflet from the Cornelia de Lange Syndrome Foundation

champion the use of particular treatments. They often find out about new advances before the busy doctor. It is easy to feel threatened in such circumstances. Ask for the information and time to digest it before responding.

Of course, some malformations are rare and have no such organisation. Parents of such children can feel left-out in the company of parents with children with more common conditions, especially if no cause has been identified. In such cases it is worth stressing that, whatever the malformation, all children's needs vary and are met on an individual basis.

The child's future

Rejection of the newborn malformed child occurs in only a minority of cases. In this situation the doctor should adopt a non-judgmental role. Rejection is more likely if the baby has been separated from the mother, a reason for avoiding unnecessary separation. Rejecting parents often state that they wish to forget all about their baby. This course can lead to severe emotional trauma manifesting even years later. Counselling should be offered on an open basis to such parents, although the offer is frequently rejected.

Parents appreciate a clear outline of the services their child will receive and express dissatisfaction if the interviewer has a lack of knowledge about medical speciality referrals or community services.[4] This problem can be overcome by preparation prior to the interview or by clearly identifying someone who will be able to give the parents all of the necessary information. This outline will include hospital medical services, community medical services, social services, and assistance from voluntary organisations. The amount of information the parents may need to absorb is large, especially if the child has multiple malformations. It is important to identify a key worker in this situation, to whom the parents can turn for advice and who can coordinate these services.

The relatives of the child will need to be told of the situation. The parents may, wish to do this themselves, but an offer to tell them by the doctor is usually taken up. If the relatives are interviewed in the presence of the parents, consistency of information is ensured, questions can be answered, misunderstandings prevented, and medical confidentiality is ensured.

Discharge

By this time the parents should have had all of their questions addressed and have a clear understanding of their child's condition and what plans have been made. It is important that the primary care team are informed and are invited to discharge planning meetings.

Many infants are subsequently readmitted to a different ward or hospital. If the parents have been given their own copy of the initial discharge summary, this can allow the admitting doctor to assimilate complex information quickly and act appropriately. Parent-held child health records of a more general nature are also useful in this regard.

Training

Training can be achieved by experience. Initially you can observe a senior colleague breaking such news and discuss key points afterwards. I and many of my colleagues appreciate having a junior member of the team in the room. They give support, ensure the information given to the parents is disseminated to the rest of the care team and they can provide useful feedback on clarity and effectiveness.

A video *Shared Concern* has been produced under the guidance of the Kings Fund Centre Informal Caring Support Unit.[12] This gives an excellent overview of the area.[13] It is accompanied by a small booklet which summarises key points, contains a list of references and also a list of voluntary organisations. The video is most useful when watched by a small group followed by a discussion.

Groups wishing to enhance their communication skills in this area can also use role play and this can include the use of professional actors taking the role of parents. Recording such consultations on videotape can then be used for detailed analysis. It is also possible to videotape real and role-played consultations for assessment of consultation skills. Reproducible and reliable instruments of assessment have been generated for analysis of such interviews,[14] although adaptation of the instrument will be required for different scenarios.

It may also be possible to arrange a visit to a nursery of infants with special needs and listen to parents reporting how the news was broken to them. The value of such direct learning has been emphasised by others.[6]

1 Wolraich ML, Siperstein GN, Reed D. Doctors' decisions and prognostications for infants with Down's syndrome. *Dev Med Child Neurol* 1991; **33**: 336-42.

2 Cooley WC, Graham ES, Moeschler JB, Graham JM. Reactions of mothers and medical professionals to a film about Down's syndrome. *Am J Dis Child* 1990;**144**:1112-6.

3 National Association for Mental Health Working Party. The birth of an abnormal child: telling the parents. *Lancet* 1971;2:1075-7.

4 Krahn GL, Hallum A, Kime C. Are there good ways to give 'bad news'? *Pediatrics* 1993;**91**:578-82.

5 Cunningham CC, Morgan PA, McGucken RB. Down's syndrome is dissatisfaction with disclosure of diagnosis inevitable? *Dev Med Child Neurol* 1984;**26**:33-9.

6 Nursey AD, Rohde JR, Farmer RD. Ways of telling new parents about their child and his or her mental handicap: a comparison of doctors' and parents' views. *J Ment Defic Res* 1991;**35**:48-57.

7 Sloper P, Turner S. Determinants of parental satisfaction with disclosure of disability. *Dev Med Child Neurol* 1993;**35**:816-25.

8 Simpson M, Buckman R, Stewart M, *et al*. Doctor-patient communication: the Toronto consensus statement. *BMJ* 1991;**303**:1385-7.

9 Ryan S. Talking to the parents of a baby who is likely to develop permanent neurological impairment following a brain insult in the perinatal period. *Postgrad Med J* 1995;**71**:336-40.
10 MacKeith R. The feelings and behaviour of parents of handicapped children. *Dev Med Child Neurol* 1973;**15**:524-7.
11 Myers BA. The informing interview: enabling parents to 'hear' and cope with bad news. *Am J Dis Child* 1983;**137**:572-7.
12 Society of Parents Helping in Education. Shared concern: breaking the news to parents that their newborn child has a disability. Informal Caring Support Unit, Kings Fund Centre, 126 Albert Street, London NW1 7NF.
13 MacManus IC, Vincent CA, Thom S, Kidd J. Teaching communication skills to clinical students. *BMJ* 1993;**306**:1322-7.
14 Cox J, Mulholland H. An instrument for assessment of videotapes of general practitioners' performance. *BMJ* 1993;**306**:1043-6.

Appendix: Useful addresses

Cornelia de Lange Syndrome Foundation UK,
'Tall Trees', 106 Lodge Lane,
Grays, Essex RM16 2RU.
Tel: 01375 376439

Down's Syndrome Association,
155 Mitcham Road, Tooting,
London SW17 9PG
Tel: 0181 682 4001

MENCAP (The Royal Society for
Mentally Handicapped Children and Adults),
MENCAP National Centre,
123 Golden Lane,
London EC1Y 0RT

Right From The Start Campaign,
c/o SCOPE,
12 Park Crescent,
London W1N 4EQ

SAFTA (Support After Termination for Abnormality),
29-30 Soho Square,
London W1V 6JB
Tel: 0171 439 6124

SOFT UK (Support Organisation for Trisomy
13/18 Related Disorders),
Tudor Lodge, Redwood,
Ross-on-Wye,
Herefordshire HR9 5UD

3 Supporting relatives following a cot death

BARBARA M PHILLIPS

Compassionate, appropriately directed support for the family of a cot death victim in the emergency department will have a profound positive effect in both the medium and long-term on the family's mourning process. In order to provide this support, the doctor needs to understand the epidemiology of the sudden infant death syndrome and to be aware of current theories of causation. This knowledge is especially important as the widespread publicity that cot death has received in the media often means that parents are well informed about risk factors and current theories. It behoves the doctor to be at least as well informed, or your ignorance will reduce the family's confidence in you. Secondly, it is important that the doctor understands the process of mourning so that it may be assisted, not impeded, in the emergency department.

Epidemiology of cot death

Most epidemiological and research studies use the term "cot death" to mean an infant found suddenly and unexpectedly dead; the term "sudden infant death syndrome" is described as a subgroup of the former in which careful postmortem examination has not revealed evidence of a fatal condition. However, some authors do use the terms interchangeably. In this article I will use the term "cot death" as we are dealing with that aspect of management which occurs before a postmortem study.

There has been a striking reduction in the incidence of cot death over the last few years both in this country and also in Holland, Australia and New Zealand. The number of cot deaths in England

Box 3.1 Cot deaths England and Wales

Year	Number
1988	1597
1989	1337
1990	1202
1991	1008
1992	531
1993	458
1994	454

and Wales from 1988 to 1994 is shown in box 3.1 (from the office of Population Censuses and Surveys). The reduction in each country appears to be related to national campaigns in which parents were given various relevant pieces of advice (box 3.2).

The UK *Back to sleep* campaign was not launched until the end of 1991 but as can be seen from box 3.1, the incidence of cot death was falling before this. There is evidence[1] that information about the hazards of prone infant sleeping was being published in magazines from the end of 1988. The *Back to sleep* campaign has certainly been subsequently associated with a further decline in the incidence of cot death. An interesting and difficult question is

Box 3.2 Advice to parents

- do not lie your baby on his or her front to sleep
- do not allow the baby to get too warm
- do not smoke in the same room as the baby
- seek early medical advice for symptoms of illness in a baby
- breast feed if possible

whether this was coincidence or whether the campaign had changed parental behaviour. There have been some studies indicating that parents are changing their babies' sleeping positions[2] but there has been little effect on the incidence of smoking. However, it is my experience that families are now aware of the dangers of passive smoking to their children's health and certainly state that their practice is no longer to smoke in the same room as their children.

With the reduced numbers of cot death following the recent campaigns, there has also been a lessening of the winter incidence peak and the age peak for babies between two to four months. The significance of these changes is unclear. There is considerable evidence demonstrating the association of cot death with poverty and smoking in the home.[3,4] The known risk factors for cot death are shown in box 3.3. Families are often aware of at least some of these and may say "It can't be a cot death because I don't smoke/he was lying on his back, etc."

Box 3.3 Risk factors of a cot death

- young maternal age
- higher parity
- winter deaths
- two to four months old
- low birth weight
- multiple births
- low social class
- smoking
- prone sleeping

Current theories of cot death causation

Although epidemiological studies show significant associations between risk factors such as prone sleeping position, prematurity and maternal smoking, they do not allow us to understand the mechanism of cot death. Parents desperately want to know why and how their baby died. These questions cannot yet be answered but there have been some useful negative studies. An obvious mechanism to explain the association between prone sleeping and cot death is the possibility that the infant suffered hypoxia or hypercapnia due to impeded breathing in this position. A review of a number of studies investigating this possibility was produced by Johnson,[5] who concluded that there was no evidence that hypoxia and hypercapnia would become significant enough to cause death in prone placed babies.

There is a large literature describing abnormalities in various organ and physiological systems in groups of infants who died from cot death compared to the results from postmortem examinations of infants dying from known causes. These include studies to show that cot death infants have an abnormal immune response with an increased number of immune cells in pulmonary tissue in one study,[6] evidence of mast cell activation suggesting a role for anaphylaxis in another[7] and evidence of increased levels of immunoglobulins in pulmonary lavage specimens.[8] Another study has shown histological abnormalities in diaphragm muscle suggesting early fatigue of the diaphragm in susceptible infants[9] and a further study has shown underdevelopment of nephrons in cot death victims' kidneys.[10] These seemingly unrelated abnormalities together suggest that infants who die from cot death may not be the completely healthy babies they had appeared. This emphasises the extreme importance of a thorough postmortem examination conducted by an experienced paediatric pathologist.

The process of mourning

It is now understood that unresolved grief can be important in the development of certain psychiatric and especially psychosomatic illnesses.[11] The effect of a cot death increases the risk for families in several aspects, including the suddenness of the death, the lack of any explanation for the death, and the fact that the death is of an infant for whom there is such expectation.

The initial reception and the management of the infant and family in the emergency department can profoundly hinder or advance the mourning process for the bereaved family. It is therefore useful that the doctor attending such a family in the immediate crisis should have an understanding of the process of mourning in order to facilitate those aspects which are germane to the crisis situation. Most workers in the field of grief and mourning have identified three or four phases through which bereaved persons pass. They may be of greater or lesser severity or length in individual persons. Psychiatric morbidity is sometimes associated with an individual's inability to pass through the various stages of grief and mourning. Engel[12] working in the 1960s, described three phases; denial and disbelief, developing awareness and, finally, resolution. Kubler-Ross, whose book *On death and dying* was the result of a long study of the mourning process, also describes similar stages of denial; rage and anger with depression and finally

---

Box 3.4 Worden's tasks of mourning

- to accept the reality of the loss
- to experience the pain of grief
- to adjust to life without the deceased person
- to "withdraw" from the deceased person and form new relationships

---

acceptance. Bowlby and Parkes (the former recognised and influential for his theories on parent-child attachment) describe an initial stage of numbness followed by pining for the lost person and disorganisation in the bereaved and finally a stage of reorganisation. As described by Couriel in *Paediatric support in sudden infant death*,[13] Worden suggested four tasks that must be undertaken by the bereaved before they can reach a state of acceptance of the death (box 3.4). The first stage of the mourning process and the first two of Worden's tasks can be facilitated or hindered in the crisis situation in the emergency department. These aspects are that the bereaved family accept the reality of their loss by having time, space and support to see, touch, hold and if they wish, to bathe and dress their dead baby. Secondly, the expression of the pain of grief can be accepted and encouraged by compassionate and supportive care from emergency department staff.

Practical aspects of care

It is usual for a warning to be received from the Ambulance Service by the emergency department informing them of the arrival of a cot death infant. It is usual for the baby to be receiving at least basic life support and in some instances advanced life support from the paramedic team. Clearly, at this stage, the situation is unknown and a diagnosis of either death or the possibility of cot death, although likely, is not clear. It is therefore appropriate for resuscitation to continue in the department's emergency room. It is often very clear that the infant is dead and has been for some time, as shown by coldness to the touch, stiffness and postmortem lividity. Under these circumstances it would not be appropriate to continue efforts at resuscitation. However, sometimes the situation is not so clear and resuscitation should continue in the usual way.

Examination/investigation of the infant

After resuscitative efforts have ceased, the infant should be thoroughly examined by a visual inspection. Note should be taken of the baby's state of nutrition and any external marks such as bruises. These should be carefully documented and distinction should be made in the documented notes between those marks known to have been caused by the resuscitative efforts, eg needle punctures and those present prior to resuscitation. Several investigations will be useful for the pathologist. These include cultures from nasopharynx, nares, stool, urine or blood. A urine obtained by suprapubic aspiration can be frozen and sent for metabolic screening. Similarly, a small skin sample can be removed and placed in culture medium. Skin cells will remain viable and can be used for the identification of inborn errors of metabolism.

However, while the investigations are extremely useful and may gain information which would otherwise be lost if the postmortem was delayed, nevertheless, individual coroners may take the view that all such investigations should be left to the pathologist. Doctors are advised not to undertake any postmortem investigations without prior agreement as to a protocol from their coroner.

Facilities for parents

Every emergency room should have a comfortably and informally furnished room for the use of distressed relatives. The room should be in or close to the "major area" of the department and it should have a pay-phone facility.

Ideally, at this stage, an experienced nurse should be assigned to the family to be a link for them during the time they remain in the emergency department. On occasions, other serious events in the department and the changing of shifts may make this very difficult but parents often express in retrospect their gratitude at having someone to explain procedures, accompany them to see their baby again and to just be there and listen at such a time.

Breaking the news

The fact that their baby is dead is often known to parents even before arriving at the hospital. However, hope often continues until a formal announcement. Even then, acceptance of the reality of death is a process requiring some time and can be much helped by the words, actions and attitudes of emergency department staff. The doctor who breaks the news to the family should be as senior as possible, ie registrar or consultant. It is important that there are no interruptions by the demands of further emergencies while the doctor is speaking with the parents.

The appearance of the doctor in the parents' room will be a signal to them that information is about to be forthcoming. There is therefore only a few seconds for the doctor to establish a caring professional relationship with the parents. Make sure that you know the parents' names and that of their baby. I have found that brief, non-invasive physical contact is helpful. Therefore I clasp each parent's hand while introducing myself and then sit down. Gentle honesty is the key to breaking the news. I usually use words such as "I am sorry to have to tell you, but despite everything we could do, your baby Jason is dead". Delivered in a sympathetic voice and with a caring manner, these words leave the parents with no lingering and confusing false hope, which may be engendered by phrases such as "Louise has slipped away". "She has gone to another place". Parents will then often turn to each other and weep. They then often start to express ideas of disbelief, confusion or anger such as "I can't believe it. She took her bottle at six o'clock". "It isn't true". "Why didn't the doctor notice something at the check-up yesterday?"

At this point, parents often want to talk about the time leading up to the discovery of the baby. This is therefore a useful time at which to take a detailed history, which is necessary for the pathological diagnosis, and to start to help the parents cope with their feelings of guilt by firmly assuring them that no action or inaction of theirs was the direct cause of the baby's death. As the history unfolds, and if the baby was clearly well or only trivially unwell over the previous two or three days, it is often appropriate to tell the parents that in your opinion it is likely that the baby has been a victim of the sudden infant death syndrome. This gives an opportunity for pointing out that a postmortem is a legal requirement and is in everyone's best interests so that any understandable cause of the baby's death can be identified. I have never known parents disturbed about the possibility of a postmortem. I think because their need to know "why?" is overwhelming. There is also a need to know "how?" Parents may express distress at the thought of their baby being unwell and them being not aware of this, or of their baby showing some symptoms that, had they been alert to, they could have attended to and thus prevented this outcome. It is therefore often appropriate to say that, in cot death, there appears to be no evidence of pain, abnormal movement or distress in the infant.

This session usually takes 20 to 25 minutes. After this time the parents have usually had answers to some of the questions and understood that others are unanswerable, certainly at this time. At this stage the parents should be invited to spend some time with their infant.

Time with the baby

As described above, the importance of the family grasping the reality of the infant's death cannot be over-emphasised. The death has been so sudden and unexpected that its unwelcome reality is difficult to internalise. Therefore, time spent with the dead infant, particularly holding and touching him, is instrumental in forwarding the healing process of mourning, although it may appear distressing to others when parents weep and have difficulty in letting go of their baby. Parents and other relatives should be encouraged to spend as much time as they wish with the baby's body. It is useful if they are initially accompanied by their nurse as there may be postmortem changes or resuscitation marks that must be explained.

It is very helpful if there can be an additional room in the emergency department where parents can spend time with their baby. In our department we have such a room between the distressed parents room and the resuscitation room and although fortunately, this is not often used, it is a great advantage.

Compassion can be shown by the emergency department staff in the presentation of the baby's body. A little crib or Moses basket with the baby's own blanket or a homely cover takes away some of the clinical appearance. The baby should be dressed in his or her own clothes (and indeed these may be necessary for forensic examination). The parents can be asked if they would like to wash and re-dress their baby in his or her own things. Parents later recall such tasks as being very beneficial to their grieving process, by making them feel they were doing what needed to be done for their infant. Clearly, this time must be parent driven and the family must not be hurried away. In some instances parents, particularly young ones, may be reluctant to see their infant. They may have hidden fears of the infant's appearance or be afraid that they will embarrass themselves by a show of emotion. These fears can be anticipated and the parents encouraged to see their infant by being told "she just looks like your baby". Sympathetic support often brings forth tears and their immediate acceptance with compassion encourages the parents to express their distress.

A similar facility should be made available to other relations. Grandparents in particular may experience extreme distress following a cot death. They have a dual grief of the death of their grandchild and their own child's distress. Furthermore, the death of a young infant while they, who may be quite elderly, continue to live again points up the "inappropriateness" of childhood death in our twentieth century society.

Older siblings of the baby, particularly those over eight or nine years old, may benefit in the same way as adults from the reality of the experience of seeing their dead baby. However, this is a sensitive area and should only be undertaken with the parents' full acceptance. Younger children have a gradually developing understanding of death, starting from the simple concept of separation. Viewing the body is probably not beneficial for younger children. However, despite their often apparent easy acceptance of their loss, young children require a great deal of reassurance and overt loving behaviour from their parents. This is because they will be experiencing their parents' distress and possibly withdrawal and also because children, particularly from the ages of four and five, may have a "magical" understanding of death whereby they may think that they have in some way harmed their infant sibling by some bad wish or thought that they had had.

Almost inevitably, the parents or other relatives will wish to return on subsequent days to see the infant again until the body is removed from the hospital. Wherever this may take place, it is important that the surroundings are made as homely and child-orientated as possible with a crib for the infant and comfortable chairs for the family.

Counsellors/religious support

Many hospitals have social workers or bereavement counsellors who provide an acute service within working hours and a follow-up support service for bereaved families. It is useful if the contact with the counsellor starts in the acute stage as practical support and advice at this time makes parents receptive to counselling from the same person at a later stage. Similarly, having ascertained the availability of the people involved, an offer of the appropriate religious support should be made.

Mementos

Occasionally, parents, when returning for further counselling sessions, express disappointment that they do not have any recent photographs of their baby. Many hospitals therefore take two or three photographs of the dead infant so that these may be given to the parents if such a request is forthcoming. Similarly, hand and foot prints or a small lock of hair would often be cherished. However, mementos should not be taken on an ad hoc basis but an agreed hospital policy should be discussed between relevant parties, including lay members of bereavement support organisations.

Going home

Sooner or later the family will want to go home. It is important that their general practitioner is informed as soon as possible so that he or she can visit the family. In the case of a breast-feeding mother the GP should be asked to prescribe a lactation-suppressing drug such as bromocriptine. The family should also be aware that once the coroner has been informed, that there is a possibility that the police may visit the scene of the infant's death, but that this is in no way an indication of any suspicion. If at all possible, no distressed person should drive the family home as this is a risk factor for a road traffic accident.

Communication

There are many people who need to be informed about the baby's death. We have found that a checklist, which can be attached to the infant's notes, reminds staff of the contacts to be made (box 3.5).

Religious observances

Different Christian denominations may emphasise different aspects at death, but in general there is no particular requirement for special handling of the body. Jewish families usually prefer

---

Box 3.5 Checklist for cot death

- child's name, date of birth, date of death
- registrar or consultant spoken to parents
- brief clinical history taken
- examination/investigations done
- parents offered to be with baby
- coroner informed
- social worker/counsellor informed
- general practitioner informed
- health visitor informed
- minister of religion contacted
- advice on registration/funeral given
- leaflet from Foundation for the Study of Infant Deaths, with telephone number of local Friends
- consultant follow-up arranged
- social worker/counsellor follow-up arranged
- community physician informed
- immunisation computer informed

---

burial to occur within 24 hours of death. This may cause a problem if the postmortem is delayed, but often pathologists are sensitive to this need and will accommodate it if possible. Muslim families may wish to undertake the preparation of the body after the postmortem but this may occur at the funeral parlour. In all cases, do not forget to enquire whether any special religious requirement is necessary and consult with the local religious leader if there is a problem.

Medium to long-term follow-up

As described earlier, because of the nature of cot death, significant medium-term distress and occasional long-term psychiatric problems are to be expected. Follow-up counselling is therefore important but is outside the scope of this chapter. A useful review is available.[13]

Staff support

Although accident and emergency department staff are not unfamiliar with sudden death, the death of an infant is always distressing. This is particularly so for staff who themselves have young infants or young grandchildren. Informal discussions allow people to express their feelings, identify good practice and feel renewed for the next occasion.

Box 3.6 Cot death research and support

The Foundation for the Study of Infant Deaths,
14 Halkin Street,
London SW1X 7DP, UK
Tel 0171 235 0965;
Cot Death Helpline 0171 235 1721;
Fax 0171 823 1986

---

1   Morley CJ. The continuing enigma of cot death. In: David TJ, ed. *Recent advances in paediatrics*, Vol 14. Edinburgh: Churchill Livingstone, 1995; pp 1-14.

2   Hiley CMH, Morley CJ. Evaluation of the government's campaign to reduce the risk of cot death. *BMJ* 1994;**309**:703-4.

3   Fleming PJ, Bacon C, Blair P, *et al*. The Confidential Enquiry into Stillbirths and Deaths in Infancy (CESDI) case control study of sudden unexpected death in infancy; I. The epidemiology of SIDS after a national risks reduction campaign. *Proc Brit Paediatr Assoc Ann Meet* 1996; Vol 68: p 86 (abstract).

4   Blair P, Fleming PJ, Bensley D, *et al*. The Confidential Enquiry into Stillbirths and Deaths in Infancy (CESDI) case control study of sudden unexpected death in infancy; III. The effects of parental smoking. *Proc Brit Paediatr Assoc Ann Meet* 1996; Vol 68: p 86 (abstract).

5   Johnson P. Infant care practices and the investigation of physiological mechanisms. *Early Hum Dev* 1994;**38**:165-79.

6   Howat WJ, Moore IE, Judd M, Roche W. Pulmonary immunopathology of sudden infant death syndrome. *Lancet* 1994;**343**:1390-2.

7   Platt MS, Yunginger JW, Sekula-Periman ST, *et al*. Involvement of mast cells in sudden infant death syndrome. *J Allergy Clin Immunol* 1994; **94**: 250-6.

8   Forsyth KD, Weeks SC, Koh L, Skinner J, Bradley J. Lung immunoglobulins in the sudden infant death syndrome. *BMJ* 1989;**298**:23-6.

9   Lamont P, Chow C, Hilton J, Pamphlett R. Differences in diaphragm fibre types in SIDS infants. *J Neuropathol Exp Neurol* 1995;**54**:32-7.

10 Siebert JR, Hass JE. Organ weights in sudden infant death syndrome. *Paediatr Pathol* 1994;**14**:973-85.

11 Worden JW. *Grief counselling and grief therapy*. New York: Springer, 1982.

12 Engel G. *Pyschological development in health and disease*. Philadelphia: WB Saunders, 1962.

13 Couriel J. Paediatric support after sudden infant death. In: David T, ed. *Recent advances in paediatrics*, Vol 9. Edinburgh: Churchill Livingstone, 1991.

4 Talking to the parents of a child in whom you suspect non-accidental or sexual abuse injury

MARION MILES

Any mention of the words child abuse gives rise to all or any of the following reactions depending on whether you are the child's parent, carer, or the professional involved: distress; disbelief; fear; denial; anger; disgust; a desire for punishment; the list is endless. Many of the reactions are common to parents and professionals and will, therefore, affect the way in which concern that abuse has taken place is discussed.

Types of abuse

Firstly we need to consider the types of abuse that occur since their different presentations require different approaches in communication. The following categories of abuse are those defined by the Department of Health in Working Together under the Children Act 1989: neglect, physical injury or non-accidental injury, sexual abuse, and emotional abuse.[1] All abuse involves some emotional ill treatment and although neglect may be acute, if, for example, a child is abandoned, it more frequently becomes apparent over a period of time. So the situations in which a doctor will most usually be required to discuss concern with a parent or carer involve physical or sexual abuse.

Why may doctors be reluctant to discuss the possibility of abuse?

In order to recognise abuse it is necessary to admit that it happens. Abuse is distasteful and shocking; it is easier, even if not consciously, to avoid considering it as a possible cause of repeated bruises, impaired growth, eating disorders, disrupted school performance or many other non-acute situations. Primary care doctors and highly focused specialists may rarely see abused children; cases that appear obvious to general and community paediatricians may not ring the right bells for their colleagues. If child abuse is rarely seen and imperfectly understood it is very difficult to discuss in any meaningful way.

Fear of removal of child from parents

Possibly the greatest cause for reluctance is concern that identifying possible abuse and thereby setting in process an enquiry by social services may result in the removal of the child from the care of the parents. Examples of dramatic dawn raids to remove children have been given great prominence by the media. The wrench of separation is undoubtedly what parents fear most. In fact only a tiny minority of parents in England lose their children at the beginning of an enquiry; research figures for 1992 suggest about 1%, or 1500 of a child population of 11 million. Even after further assessment and conference only another 3000 children enter care against their parents' wishes. A further 3000 are voluntarily accommodated. Wider knowledge of these figures should reassure parents and professionals alike whilst not minimising the potential distress for individual families.

Litigation

Doctors are becoming more aware of litigation. A wrong, even if very well motivated, diagnosis of possible sexual abuse may not be accepted as such. Assaults on doctors are increasing and nightmares of being waylaid by an angry parent are common even if not borne out in reality.

Confidentiality

The issues surrounding confidentiality are complex. They make many doctors reluctant to participate in child protection work, let alone share information with a social services colleague. The Children Act 1989 embodies the principle that the welfare of a child is the paramount consideration.[2] However all doctors have a legal and ethical duty to maintain confidentiality, and should not disclose information without consent unless disclosure can be justified by serving the best interest of the child.

Conflict of interests

For family practitioners, who may be involved with the alleged abusers as well as the abused child and other family members, there may appear to be a conflict of interests. This understandable concern can be resolved by meeting the child's best interests.

Who communicates with whom?

When child abuse or neglect is suspected, the doctor is usually required to share relevant information with a statutory agency responsible for child protection (the statutory agencies are social services, NSPCC and the police). When a critical threshold of professional concern has been reached a referral to a statutory agency *must* be made. However when the situation is uncertain the doctor may communicate with a colleague or senior social worker for advice.

Under a recent departmental document *Child Protection: Clarification of Arrangements Between the NHS and other Agencies,* units and trusts are required to identify a named professional for child protection who is able to provide advice and support. These named professionals in turn relate to the senior designated doctor, identified by the health authority, who has health authority-wide responsibilities and is a member of the Area Child Protection Committee (ACPC). Further guidance as to how to consult and obtain advice should be clearly laid out in local ACPC guidelines. When passing on sensitive information the doctor needs to consider the likely consequences of its being shared or not. Doctors must take care to avoid guaranteeing confidentiality, especially when a child or young person has disclosed abuse. The time scale within which communication is taking place should also be considered. Information may be more appropriately shared during day working hours when experienced colleagues are more readily available; however in some situations information may need to be shared more urgently to ensure protection from further injury.

Next, it is important to consider who else needs to be informed and what information should be shared. Information held by health visitors and school nurses, for example, may assume a different significance after consultation. Similarly a past history of violence or child molestation may surface following contact with social services or the police, and give a different emphasis to the original concern.

Doctors need to be able to go beyond the words offered but also listen to innuendos and inferences behind the words, in order to develop better communication skills. Observation of body language may modify the words used or prompt the doctor to pursue further specific details. The doctor needs to ask why certain information is being given; for example, a mother may report that her baby is crying excessively and this worries her partner. Does she mean the baby is being shaken and she wants a careful examination? Is *she* feeling very stressed herself, and so worried that she might lose control that she attributes the threat of abuse to her partner? When she reports that her 6 year old daughter now refuses to be minded by Mr Jones next door is she expressing irritation or fear of sexual abuse? If a reported story suggests abuse a careful documentation of what was actually said, together with the possible interpretations and details of any proposed action, is essential.

Why do we need to communicate well?

In the foreword to a recent publication, *Child Protection Messages from Research*,[6] there is an important acknowledgement that we must not pretend that actions taken by child protection agencies can guarantee that parents will not harm their children. This is important because it should stop social workers becoming scapegoats and reduce the undertaking of draconian measures in order to avoid criticism. It should also encourage the community at large to take more responsibility in the prevention of abuse rather than leaving it to the professionals.

Communicating with parents

The Children Act supports greater parental involvement by the development of services encouraging parents and professionals to

41

work in partnership in order to meet the needs of their children. In the context of child protection, where this balance has been finely tuned, research shows that outcomes are better and social work made easier when parents are involved in the process throughout. Cleaver and Freeman[3] highlighted the way in which families feel invaded and humiliated by the investigation of possible abuse. When not involved from the outset the family structures suffered. Clearly it is essential to communicate concern rather than critical confrontation.

A review of child protection cases by Thoburn, Lewis and Shemmings[4] asked parents and carers if they were kept informed of what was happening; just under 50% said they were not. In over half of those cases where continuing communication was good, the outcome (judged by specific criteria) was also judged to be good. Parents, whether implicated in abuse or not, felt a better job had been done when they were listened to and talked to by the professionals. Parents as citizens have rights to know what is said about them; children and young people have specific rights to information under the UN Convention on the Rights of the Child. Good, sensitive communication skills are necessary in order to fulfil these obligations.

Communicating with children

As far as the children caught up in abusive situations are concerned, they too value highly sensitive communication. They expect privacy and do not always understand the limits on confidentiality. The older ones are painfully aware that their disclosure of abuse may result in fragmentation of their families. Along with a desire for justice, there may be feelings of guilt at the result. Children sometimes face criticism and, in the case of sexual abuse, allegations of encouragement. Poor self image and low self esteem may result in eating disorders, rebellion or promiscuity. Specialist support may be indicated, but a few sensitive words of praise, when a child first discloses, and reassurance that being abused does not mean they are bad, will go a long way to prevent a feeling of worthlessness.

The majority (at least 70%) of child protection conferences are now attended throughout or for a large part of the time by the parents of the child in whom abuse is suspected. This development ensures clarity about the allegation of abuse, provides a forum where findings are shared, and allows parents (and children when appropriate) to contribute and perhaps correct misinformation. Since the family members will hear about a doctor's concern either directly or in a written report it is highly desirable that the information presented has already been shared with them by the doctor concerned. All health information should be readily comprehensible and not made opaque by medical jargon. It should also be strictly relevant to child protection issues and not descend into a rambling account of family health.

What do you say and to whom?

When required to discuss concern about possible abuse, it is important to ensure that you are doing so with a parent who has parental responsibility. A mother has parental responsibility by right but her partner may not, even if he is the father. Until recently many doctors faced with injuries or other symptoms and signs suggestive of child abuse have faltered in sharing their concerns and conclusions with parents or carers. They may fear that further abuse will be a consequence or that the parent will take offence and disappear. In fact there is little evidence that this happens.

For reasons given earlier family practitioners often find themselves in more difficult situations than, say, a paediatrician who can more easily keep the child's best interests foremost in mind. For whatever reason it is tempting to be non-committal to the parent and to contact social services as the statutory agency in the expectation that they will deal with the concern. Clearly this is poor practice: the truth will out at a conference and research confirms that the majority of families, however angry at the time, prefer professionals to be "up front" and not to go behind their backs!

No one pretends that it is easy to tell a parent that child abuse is suspected but, initially at any rate, it is rarely necessary to be confrontational. It is acceptable to explain that the injuries displayed are not those usually seen in the circumstances described: the advice of a hospital colleague is indicated to see what might be the true cause. A wary parent may at this point say "do you think this is abuse?", to which the honest reply is "I don't know but we must find out what has happened to see if treatment is necessary". Parents respond positively to professional concern. It may even provide an opportunity for the parent to say "I'm worried he (the child) might have been hit or shaken" and name a

43

specific suspect. Parents are usually overly anxious about their babies so a recommendation to see a specialist is rarely dismissed. Clearly if there is concern that the child's life is at immediate risk the doctor will have to be more explicit, explain the need to involve social services and, if necessary, arrange for a specialist examination. Involvement of the police to ensure the child's safety may, on rare occasions, be indicated. In less clear cut situations there may be concern about the parent-child relationship, a suggestion of ill treatment, behavioural problems, or poor growth.

In these and similar circumstances a consultation rather than an urgent referral to social services is appropriate, once the parent is aware of the range of support and advice that is available through this agency. Consultation with the local designated doctor or other paediatrician may also be helpful.

A sensitive approach and careful choice of words is always essential, taking account of differing family lifestyles and child rearing practices. These consultations should not be hurried and benefit from being undertaken in privacy. The language used by the family must be considered, but without using family members as interpreters. Young people may seek advice the nature of which raises concern of possible abuse. You must not give a promise of confidentiality while seeking ways of providing support which does not contribute further to the abuse.

Once abuse is no longer merely suspected but more certain after investigation, the situation is equally challenging. The only possible justification for confrontation in the early stages of an enquiry may be when injuries and other findings can be explained in no other way. Currently our aim is to identify children in need in order to support families so that they can continue to care for their children. Previously the emphasis was on confrontational investigation following allegation on suspicion of abuse. This is stressful for families and professionals alike and serves to alienate families from the care and support of their children.

If the identification of children in need is done sensitively and with the involvement of other caring agencies, our communication skills will have been used to good effect.

Do we agree what abuse is?

There are wide ranging views about what constitutes child abuse, and it is important to be aware of these in order to be able to advise about it convincingly. Broken bones do not usually give rise to debate but to prevent a light tap becoming a severe beating parents need to be counselled sympathetically rather than judgmentally.

The attitudes and views of different ethnic and cultural groups may be affected by their customs and religious beliefs, and it is essential to understand these issues, while bearing in mind the best interests of the child. What is considered normal behaviour in different families varies considerably; similarly what concerns families may not concern professionals. A study by Smith and Grocke[5] showed that masturbation, which may be considered an indication of abuse, occurred in 67% of apparently normal families. Bathing with parents, which may also concern professionals, occurred in 77% of the families studied.

Where do you learn the necessary skills?

Doctors in training will benefit from sitting in with a senior doctor during discussions on possible child abuse with a parent. Junior doctors should never have to confirm abuse with a parent but should, from the beginning, understand the need to keep parents informed during the process. Attendance at child protection conferences also provides a good model as to how to communicate with parents in these circumstances.

Training sessions organised on behalf of the ACPC provide opportunities to engage in role play and thereby refine your communication skills.

In conclusion, the communication skills required in this situation reflect those needed in general. Contact with the relevant named professional and designated doctors is recommended in order to know where to get specific advice. It is also helpful to be familiar with the local ACPC guidelines.

1 Department of Health. *Working together under the Children Act 1989.* London: HMSO, 1991.
2 Department of Health. *An introduction to the Children Act.* London: HMSO, 1989.
3 Cleaver H, Freeman P. *Parental perspectives in cases of suspected child abuse.* London: HMSO, 1995.
4 Thoburn J, Lewis A, Shemmings D. *Paternalism or partnership.* London: HMSO, 1995.
5 Smith M, Grocke M. *Normal family sexuality and sexual knowledge in children.* London: Royal College of Psychiatrists, Gorkill Press, 1995.
6 Department of Health. *Child protection: message from research.* London: HMSO, 1995.

5 Your child is brain dead

ALASTAIR W BLAIR, CHRISTOPHER R STEER

The daunting situation of dealing with brain death, with the implied requirement to decide whether continuation of life support is appropriate, is a relatively uncommon challenge in paediatrics. However, with the advent of increasingly sophisticated intensive care, this problem arises sufficiently frequently to mean that most paediatricians in acute hospital practice will be confronted with it at intervals during their professional careers. The literature suggests that 1% of neonates who die are determined "brain dead" and that in paediatric intensive care units, between 1% and 2% of admissions eventually fulfil the criteria for brain death.[2-5] Ischaemic anoxic insults and brain trauma account for more than two-thirds of brain deaths in paediatric intensive care units (box 5.1).[5]

Box 5.1 Aetiology of brain death in paediatric intensive care units[5]

ischaemic anoxic insults	41%*
CNS trauma	32%*
infections	10%
cerebrovascular disease	8%
metabolic	6%
structural	3%
n	387**

*Particularly when combined in child abuse
**66% aged under 5 years

What is brain death?

Brain death may be defined as irreversible loss of function of the whole brain.[6-9] Absent cerebral cortical and brainstem function are regarded as constituting the death of the individual. Irreversible absence of all brainstem functions is the cornerstone of diagnosis in brain death.[7,10,11] Since loss of lower brainstem function implies loss of the capacity to breath spontaneously, brain death can only be "observed" in patients undergoing artificial ventilation. Because of the need for viable whole organs for transplantation, criteria are therefore required for brain death which allow physicians to perform tests to fulfil those criteria while the patient (potential donor) is haemodynamically stable with organs which are in an optimal condition for transplantation. The well known Harvard criteria were first drawn up in 1968[10] and were designed to determine "whole" brain death, including death of the neocortex, ie, excluding the persistent vegetative state. These original criteria have been extensively discussed and modified for use in paediatric practice[1,12-15] and, in spite of some controversy, particularly with regard to assessment of brain death in neonates, a consensus approach to the determination of brain death in children has been generally agreed[5,16-18] The criteria for determination of brain death in children are summarised in box 5.2.

Preparing the ground

Progress of a child towards brain death can sometimes be anticipated and in this situation it may be useful to help the parents realise the gravity of the situation before pronoucement of brain death is actually made. Even when the diagnosis is clinically evident to attending medical staff, it is sometimes appropriate to allow time to pass so that the parents realise for themselves, possibly assisted by discussions with the nursing and medical staff, the reality of the situation. Sufficient length and depth of relationship between the attending professionals and parents is helpful in assisting relatives to cope with a tragic experience that none of them will ever forget. When time is available, this allows exploration of the beliefs and faiths of parents and may help to identify which agencies in the community they are likely to turn to, or find acceptable, in the aftermath, when formal contact with the intensive care unit will have ceased. Time also helps to generate a degree of mutual respect upon which mutual support can be

---

Box 5.2 Brain death guidelines in children (modified from[16])

The examination should be carried out by two physicians:

History: determine the cause of coma to eliminate remediable or reversible conditions eg, drug effects; hypothemia, metabolic disorders; surgically remediable brainstem compression

Physical examination:

● coma and apnoea
● absent brainstem function

  ● mid position or fully dilated pupils
  ● absent oculocephalic "doll's eye" movement
  ● absent caloric-induced eye movement
  ● absent corneal, gag, cough, suck and root reflexes
  ● absent respiratory movement with standardised testing for apnoea
  ● patient not hypothermic or hypotensive
  ● flaccid tone and absent spontaneous or induced movement (excluding reflex, spinal flex or activity)
  ● consistent examination findings throughout a predetermined period of observation

Suggested period and investigation according to age:

● up to 2 months: two examinations with isoelectric EEGs 48 hours apart
● 2 months and over: two examinations 12–24 hours apart depending on age with corroborative EEG (electrocerebral silence) if possible and where feasible radionucleotide scanning or cerebroangiography demonstrating absent cerebral flow★

★For more detailed discussion of age-dependent examination techniques and role of ancillary tests see refs 5 and 19

---

based. This mutuality of support is important because intensive care staff often suffer considerable stress in these situations and parents may themselves play an enormously important role (sometimes unwittingly) in helping staff to cope.

Families, of course, vary considerably in how they react to these situations; for example, grandparents or other members of a wider family can be brought into the process by parents and may be of great value in helping them to approach issues which they find difficult to confront. Formal meetings with parents form an important part of information giving and gathering, for example, planned meetings with the consultant who has overall responsibility for a child's care. These meetings are probably best regarded as "way points" in a continuing process of contact with the intensive care unit professionals. It is obviously necessary that parts of the process such as disclosing the diagnosis of brain death, and deciding whether to continue life support should be a more formal, and duly recorded and witnessed process; but the continuum of contact will identify those people within the professional team to whom the parents relate best.

Facing the issue

Once the diagnosis of brain death has been realised, the obvious next issue is whether to continue or discontinue life support. If this is delayed for too long and there is any question of organ donation for transplantation purposes, organ viability may suffer as a result of loss of homeostasis which accompanies brain death.[5] Many parents will arrive at their own decision regarding life support unprompted but in any case it is wiser to "stage-manage" the process so that the parents are allowed to arrive at their own decision on the matter whilst feeling that they are taking the initiative. Even though some will turn to professionals for their support and advice it is important to remember that in future years these same parents will go over the decision-making processes in their minds again and again. It is crucial for them to feel that they were in no way pressurised. In determining the final decision

---

Case history 5.1

Hearsay from other cases

Parents report they have heard of comatose cases on life-support systems for long periods of time eventually making full recovery.

Reassurances:

- these cases are persistent vegetative state which, if looked into in detail, would not fulfil the present criteria of brain death
- some of these anecdotal examples date back to the controversies that led to definition of brain death, and still circulate
- a great deal of account has to be taken of the matter of irreversibility, particularly prompted by the need to make organ donation acceptable. There is therefore more professional conviction that the criteria are satisfactory

---

whether to discontinue life support the parental decision is obviously paramount and takes precedence.

The second point is to support parents in whichever decision they make. If they agree that life support should be discontinued then it is of fundamental importance that they should be absolutely convinced that the child *is* brain dead and they should, therefore, have the matter explained to them in detail and should be encouraged to ask any questions or even witness any of the testing personally. This is time well spent because the agonies of doubt which may assail parents who feel that they may have made the decision too hastily must be hard to bear. There are reports of patients recovering from persistent vegetative states after prior periods of life support. These must be very disturbing to parents who have elected to discontinue such life support and it is therefore important to explain clearly the difference between ventilator-dependent brain dead individuals and those who are in a persistent vegetative state. The natural tendency to spare parents' sensitivities by using euphemisms and not fully including them in the very stressful process of switching off, is misguided. Their questions must be answered sensitively but factually. They must be allowed time for reflection and any re-iteration of the questioning should be accepted sympathetically.

Once the decision is taken to discontinue life support it should not be implemented with undue haste and the parents should be

---

Case history 5.2

Differing view between parents

A couple agree to proceed to "switch off" their dead infant but senior nursing staff report suspicion that father wants this and mother agrees verbally but seems unhappy and unconvinced.

Suggested action:

- senior decision maker meets couple together and re-iterates the ground
- emphasis is on **not** to rush or pressurise the decision
- opportunity is sought to confront the issue of non-concordance of view and implications discussed
- offer opportunity of other counselling agencies
- indicate the undesirability of acting until unanimity reached
- fix a review of the situation after a short interval

allowed time to decide, after consultation with the wider family if desired, how they wish it to be effected. Some will wish the involvement of religious ceremonies and some may wish independent counselling; such things are usually possible to arrange in the circumstances. At the stage of managing the switching off process, some may wish to be present, some may not. At this juncture the clinician in charge of the case must give due consideration to the other staff working in the unit who may themselves require some support. In general it should be the most senior person available who actually turns the switches. For the purposes of higher medical training it may be necessary and desirable for other members of the junior or middle grade staff to be present in order to witness and learn from the process. Delegation of a "switching off" task to junior staff is inappropriate and is best avoided wherever possible.

Continuation of cardiac impulses after switches have been turned off can be found by some to be quite distressing. Parents and less experienced staff should be given due warning about this; continuing a visible and audible ECG monitor is usually inappropriate where auscultation will suffice to determine asystole. In the case of children, many parents will wish the child to die in their arms and the life support systems can be disconnected for this purpose, along with the monitoring equipment. Due attention must be given to the degree of privacy which is appropriate for parents in this phase of acute grief. Experienced nursing staff are invaluable in giving appropriate weight to this kind of detail. Side-room accommodation is obviously ideal, but where this is not available consideration has to be given to such matters as the number of the professional attendants present in the room at the time of death, the possibility that there may be visitors to other children in the unit and the intrusion by clinical routines being carried out nearby.

Should the parents decide against discontinuation of life support, the immediate process of decision-making is postponed but the overall situation is, if anything, rather more difficult to manage. As mentioned above, the clinician's duty is to support the parents in their decision and not to try and influence it otherwise. It is quite likely that they will finally arrive at the decision to switch off at a later date and there is no way of anticipating when that point will be reached.

Immediate provision following death must allow parents an

expression of acute grief in private or in the company of the people they request to be present. An appropriate quiet room or area should be identified for this beforehand; experienced nursing staff are usually particularly helpful and thoughtful with regard to practical issues, such as providing tea and tissues at this stage and are often less reticent than many medical staff in providing direct emotional support. Effectiveness in breaking bad news and dealing with distressed relatives is something that improves with experience. Increasingly, however, these skills can be improved by teaching, eg, using video or role-play. The literature contains some useful pointers,[20-24] and for example, explores such issues as non-verbal communication and the role of touch.[25-27] "Non-touching" is described as the "English disease".[27]

It seems harsh that in this phase parents are likely to be asked to give their permission for a postmortem examination, although this will be easier for them if the matter has been the subject of discussion beforehand. It is important to most parents that the availability of contact with the professionals in the intensive care unit is not simply "turned off" at this point. They need to know that the people who have been expressing concern and support

---

Box 5.3 Aftermath

- identify an appropriate time and place for acute grief
- emotional and related care needs of family's other children to be catered for by involving minister, priest, rabbi or social agency to provide emotional support and comfort
- involve primary care team—general practitioner, health visitor
- follow-up visits, eg, to discuss outstanding issues, postmortem reports, etc.
- care, counselling and support of medical and nursing team

---

really *do* care about their child and about the outcome (such seemingly trivial matters as, for example, what happens to the child's favourite toys is of help). Parents may develop acute anxieties about some particular question, logical or illogical, and wish to speak to senior medical or nursing staff to have their anxieties alleviated. This should be done by the most expeditious means possible, eg, by telephone or an informal follow-up visit, without the delays implied by a need to make appointments, etc.

Longer term support

A formal follow-up appointment may be a useful means of allowing parents to bring up any questions or comments that may linger in their minds and to discuss the postmortem results. Many parents will have found their own source of support without the hospital, but it is useful to have some information about bereavement and counselling services offered either at interview or in the form of a pamphlet. It is appropriate to raise this subject with them at some point as many parents will feel inhibited to

---

Box 5.4 Some "do nots"

- do not rush or pressurise a decision
- do not become impatient with request to cover the same ground many times
- do not withhold information
- do not peripheralise the parents in the decision process
- do not over-promote the issue of organ donation
- do not withdraw contact after the "switch off"

Box 5.5 Summary points

- establish brain death with *certainty* using recognised criteria
- prepare and discuss with parents/family
  - the underlying condition
  - what constitutes brain death
  - why and how it has occurred
  - differences between brain death and persistent vegetative state
- provide emotional and practical support—continual contact between the family and
  - a responsible decision maker
  - the intensive care staff providing hour by hour care
- allow time for acceptance of the situation
- involve the parents centrally in final decision making and participation in the "switch off" process if requested
- when counselling sit close enough to be easily seen and heard in an area where you won't be disturbed; avoid physical barriers such as tables or desks; achieve and sustain eye contact; extend a comforting touch to the relative's shoulder or hand, if appropriate.

53

make the contact on their own initiative, but will accept the offer of help from people they know to put them in touch. The general practitioner should always be informed and may play a key role in supporting the family. If there is evidence of a prolonged or maladaptive grieving process either in parents or siblings of the dead child, counselling and psychology follow up services may be required.

Ultimate overall management comprises a combination of common sense, sensitivity and compassion on the part of medical and nursing staff dealing with these tragic situations. With attention to detail and careful planning the process can be made less painful for all concerned, with an emphasis on an understanding and positive approach rather than one is either "blunt and unfeeling" or "kind and sad".[22,23] Historically education of nursing and medical staff in this area has been on an "apprenticeship" basis through experience rather than formal teaching and in some cases junior staff have been placed in inappropriate situations of managing brain death. There is some evidence that the education needs of undergraduate and postgraduate students in this area are now beginning to be addressed.[28-32]

Many units are also developing follow-up counselling and support groups for medical and nursing staff to help them cope with the processes outlined above. Such critical incident "debriefing"[32] is certainly desirable and necessary, particularly in paediatric intensive care units with a high patient turnover. This helps to minimise chronic anxiety and burn-out in staff and promotes the concept of team work which is so vital in the management of sick children and their families. Some of the points discussed above are summarised in boxes 5.3 and 5.5.

1   Ashwal S, Schneider S. Brain death in the newborn. *Paediatrics* 1989;**84**:429-37.
2   Edmonds JF, Wong S. Paediatric brain death and organ transplantation. In: Kaufman HH, ed. *Pediatric brain death and organ/tissue retrieval: medical, ethical and legal aspects.* New York: Plenum Publishing Corp. 1989; p89.
3   Bruce D. Brain death in children: the Philadelphia experience. In: Kaufman HH, ed. *Pediatric brain death and organ/tissue retrieval: medical, ethical and legal aspects.* New York: Plenum Publishing Corp. 1989; p83.
4   Black PM, Torres ID. Brain death in children: guidelines and experience at the Massachusetts General Hospital. In: Kaufman HH, ed. *Pediatric brain death and organ/tissue retrieval: medical, ethical and legal aspects.* New York: Plenum Publishing Corp. 1989; p75.
5   Ashwal S, Schneider S. Paediatric brain death: current perspectives. *Adv Pediatr* 1991;**38**:181-202.

6   A definition of irreversible coma: Report of the Ad Hoc Committee of the Harvard Medical School to examine the definition of brain death. *JAMA* 1968;**205**:337.

7   An appraisal of the criteria of cerebral death: a summary statement. *JAMA* 1976; **237**: 982.

8   Conference of the Royal Colleges and Faculties of the United Kingdom. Diagnosis of brain death. *Lancet* 1976;2:1069.

9   Report of the Medical Consultants on the diagnosis of death to the Presidents Commission for the Study of Ethical Problems in Medicine and Biomedical and Behavioural Research: Guidelines for the determination of brain death. *Neurology* 1982;**32**:395-9.

10 Black PM. Brain death. *N Engl J Med* 1978;**299**:393-400.

11 Ad Hoc Committee on Brain Death, The Childrens Hospital Boston. Determination of brain death. *J Pediatrics* 1987;**110**:15-9.

12 Volpe JJ. Commentary. Brain death determination in the newborn. *Pediatrics* 1987;**80**:293-7.

13 Coulter DL. Special article. Neurologic uncertainty in newborn intensive care. *N Engl J Med* 1986;**316**:840-4.

14 Watchko JF. Neurologic uncertainty in newborn intensive care. *N Engl J Med* 1987;**317**:960.

15 Ashwal S. Brain death in the newborn. *Clin Perinatal* 1989; **16**: 501-8.

16 Guidelines for the determination of brain death in children. *Pediatrics* 1987;**80**:298-300.

17 Stephenson C. Brain death in children. *Focus Crit Care* 1987; **14**: 49-56.

18 Moshe SL, Alvarez LA. Diagnosis of brain death in children. *J Clin Neurophysiol* 1986;**3**:239-49.

19 Farrell MM, Levin DL. Brain death in the pediatric patient: historical, sociological, medical, religious, cultural, legal and ethical considerations. *Crit Care Med* 1933;**21**:1951-65.

20 Campbell ML. Breaking bad news to patients - clinical guidelines. *JAMA* 1994;**271**:1052.

21 McLaughlan CAJ. Handling distressed relatives and breaking bad news. *BMJ* 1990;**301**:1145-9.

22 Charlton RC. Breaking bad news. *Med J Aust* 1992; **157**: 615.

23 Brewin TR. Three ways of giving bad news. *Lancet* 1991; **337**: 1207-9.

24 Kaiser RMM. The challenge of breaking bad news. (editorial). *Hosp Pract* 1993;**28**:13-4.

25 Breaking bad news - knowledge for practice - professional development. *Nursing Times* 1994;**90**:(suppl) 1-4.

26 Buis C, De Boo T, Hull R. Touch and breaking bad news. *Fam Pract* 1991;**8**:303-4.

27 Heylings PNK. Personal View. *BMJ* 1973;2:111.

28 Sykes N. Medical students fears about breaking bad news. *Lancet* 1989;2(8662):564.

29 Knox JDE, Thomson GM. Breaking bad news: medical undergraduate communication skills teaching and learning. *Med Educ* 1989;**23**:258-61.

30 Pearce P. Breaking bad news. *Med J Aust* 1993;**158**:137.

31 Charlton RC. Letter in reply to Bruyn NJ. Breaking bad news. *Med J Aust* 1993;**158**:137-8.

32 Gillard JH, Dent THS, Aarons E, *et al*. Preregistration house officers in the Thames Regions: changes in the quality of training after four years. *BMJ* 1993;**307**:1176-9.

33 Swanson RW. Psychological issues in CPR. *Ann Emerg Med* 1993;**22**:350-3.

COMMUNICATION SKILLS IN MEDICINE

Appendix: some useful addresses

"SANDS"

Stillbirth and Neonatal Death Society,
28 Portland Place,
LONDON W1N 4DE
Helpline: 0171 436 5881
Publications: 0171 436 7940
Fax: 0171 436 3715
Local group contact numbers should be available at every maternity unit. Self-help and support in stillbirth and neonatal deaths. (Each hospital should have contact arrangements for their own Regional Transplant Co-ordinator, who usually offers counselling and follow up arrangements directly or via other agencies.)

Compassionate Friends

6 Denmark Street,
BRISTOL BS1 5DQ
Tel: 0117 929 2778

Nationwide network for self help for bereaved parents

British Organ Donor Society (Body)

Balsham,
CAMBRIDGE CB1 6DL
TEL: 01223 893636

Self help and support on organ donation issues

CRUSE (For Care of the Bereaved)

CRUSE House,
126 Skene Road,
Richmond
SURREY TW9 1UR
Tel: 0171 940 4818

6 Communicating with young adults with cystic fibrosis

ANTHONY K WEBB

Introduction

The future for young adults with cystic fibrosis (CF) is slowly being transformed by scientific breakthroughs and medical expertise into one of better survival and improved quality of life. Three decades ago, the majority of CF patients died as children and the burden of care and knowledge of the disease was the responsibility of the parents. Expert paediatric care has produced a growing population of young CF adults which, by the year 2000, will number 3000 in the UK. This will be equal to the number of paediatric patients. Mean actuarial survival is now into the third decade of life,[1] and it is anticipated that CF babies born today will survive into the fourth decade of life.[2] This enormous burden of care, previously the responsibility of parents, is now being transferred to the young adults. Adolescents will be faced with complex issues such as deciding whether to have a transplant or perhaps understanding the current state of gene therapy.

Despite increasing optimism, CF remains a lethal disease. Nearly all patients will die from pulmonary sepsis unless they receive an organ transplant. This ultimate treatment only increases survival by a mean of three years for 50% of recipients. The ability to communicate well with a group of young people who have a limited future but desire to lead a normal life in a competitive world is not an easy undertaking. Knowledge on the part of the carer of the multiple needs of these young adults will improve the ability to communicate. Understanding their anxieties and fears

> **Box 6.1 Why young CF adults are different from their peers**
>
> - they have a lethal illness
> - all men are sterile
> - poor body image due to poor nutritional status
> - they have considerable medical knowledge
> - CF friends will have died of the same disease from which they will eventually die
> - they have an enormous burden of daily self-care
> - difficulties in getting mortgages, life insurances and employment when life tables show mean survival only into the third decade of life
> - CF will have a considerable impact on family life and family dynamics

and providing reassurance will enhance communication. Some of the important areas of interaction between CF patients and carers are discussed in this chapter.

Understanding young adults with CF

Limited life-expectancy

Several factors differentiate CF adolescents from their healthy peers (box 6.1). Perception of a limited future leads some patients deliberately to lead a life in the fast lane. Recurrent speeding offences, participation in high-risk adventure sports such as parachuting and bungi jumping, and also experimentation with recreational drugs are often a feature of a CF lifestyle. However, despite the differences, patients with CF do lead remarkably normal lives until the terminal stages of the illness. A recent survey showed that 54% were employed and 30% of the remainder were students.[3] Approximately 30% of CF adults are married or in long term relationships. Despite the burden of a potentially lethal disease, the majority of CF adults function psychosocially at the same level as their healthy peers.[4,5] The process by which CF adults cope is probably to minimise to themselves, their peers and close partners the degree of severity of their disease. This is reflected in one study where individual patients described themselves as healthier than other CF adults.[6] A recent study extended this precept and found that CF adults and their close companions underestimated disease severity and overestimated self-care when compared to the evaluation of their physician.[7] This mechanism of coping with daily living is useful but causes communication difficulties when disease progression breaches this defence, and the patient is confronted with preterminal care and the need for transplantation.

Medical problems

The adolescent with CF has formidable medical problems. Most adolescents are transferred to continuing adult care when 16-18 years old. They may also be leaving home and losing family support. At this time, they also become responsible for their own care. The demands of their daily self-care are time consuming (box 6.2). Compliance with self-care and coping with a potentially lethal disease may totally determine lifestyle just as they are trying to achieve normality. Conversely, changes in lifestyle may also determine disease progression if they have detrimental effect upon self-care.

Box 6.2 Daily timetable of self-care in a young CF patient

Functions	am (min)	pm (min)	total (min)
physiotherapy	20	20	40
nebulised drugs (bronchodilators, antibiotics, DNase)	20	20	40
exercise	15	15	30
total	55	55	110

All patients will take considerable amounts of oral medication; and those with diabetes will take insulin and monitor control

Sicker patients may use enteral feeding and require non-invasive nocturnal ventilation

---

Self-knowledge

The majority of CF adults have considerable knowledge of their disease. They have grown up with the illness and many of their friends will have died from it. They communicate with each other through their own national and international meetings. They publish their own national and international journals which are as informed as any medical journal. Consequently they are often extremely knowledgeable of the minutiae of the disease and current scientific advances. It should also be emphasised that not all CF patients are knowledgeable and some are woefully ignorant or slow to absorb information about the disease. Carers will need to take such variations into account and adapt their style of communication accordingly.

Comprehensive knowledge in the majority of patients can place those carers who are still learning about the disease at a considerable disadvantage. This principle applies especially to junior doctors, nurses, and physiotherapists in training who rotate through a specialist CF unit to receive education about the disease. These junior staff may have difficulties in communicating and giving advice to CF patients who are the same age, have the same interests and are going to die. It is also important for them not to assume an arrogant or defensive approach to an ebullient and informed young CF patient. Burnout in CF carers who become too emotionally involved is also a well recognised phenomenon.

Who communicates with CF patients?

CF is a complicated, multisystem, disease. Care of CF patients requires a multidisciplinary input (box 6.3). This is best delivered, as recommended, from specialist centres.[8,9] Preference has been expressed by the majority of CF patients[10] that their care is received in specialist centres. Patient survival is better in those units which have experience and have developed expertise appropriate to the speciality.[11] A team approach allows the individual patient to

---

Box 6.3 Members of a multidisciplinary CF team

- doctors
- physiotherapists
- dieticians
- social workers
- nurses (ward and community)
- secretaries
- medical students

---

communicate about specific problems with a CF expert such as a dietician, social worker, physiotherapist or doctor. Communication is a two-way process. The ability to communicate will vary for different carers and patients and success will depend upon the ability to establish a rapport. Negotiating the balance of treatment may result in a compromise acceptable to both patient and carer which, in medical terms, may be considered insufficient. The care of in-patients with severe disease may be more complicated, communication and education become more intense and are best delivered in the environment of a dedicated CF ward.

Common discussion topics between CF adults and carers

Some of the commoner areas of repeated discussion where good communication is essential are discussed below (box 6.4). Time will often have to be set aside from the routine out-patient visit to encompass some of these difficult topics.

Box 6.4 Common discussion topics between CF adults and carers

- transition from paediatric to adult care
- reproduction
- self-care, education and compliance
- transplantation
- the future

Transition from paediatric to adult care

The period of time when the young adolescent transfers from paediatric to adult care is of crucial importance. If the receiving CF adult unit fails to establish a good rapport with the new patient it may take a long time to correct the damage. When the young adolescent leaves the paediatric unit, several changes are occurring at once. Parental care is being relinquished and transferred to patient self-care. It is important, however, to retain links and communication with the family who have supported the patient for so long. Later, as disease progression occurs, the patient will need to renew this bonding.

The ability to fulfil the rigours of daily self-care will depend upon the maturity of the patient. Questioning previously held

61

views is a feature of this phase. Often the adolescent may be undergoing a rebellious phase, totally independent of the disease. Self-care may be abandoned. It is not uncommon for medical deterioration to accelerate during adolescence. Carers may need to respond sensitively to the wish of patients to have greater control.

It is extremely important for the paediatric unit to prepare the child for transfer to an adult clinic. Some paediatric and adult units achieve this by holding joint transition clinics. It is easier for patients to transfer to a well-established adult clinic when their adult peers have preceded them and passed back favourable opinions through the grapevine.

Reproductive issues

Part of leading a normal life for CF adults is to have long-term relationships and many would like a family. Unfortunately all the men are sterile and choosing the best time to impart this information to a young adolescent requires great sensitivity. Often, the men find out incidentally from booklets or other patients.

Women with CF are as fertile as the normal population. Contraception should be discussed with them routinely by medical staff. Pregnancy should only be recommended to women with good respiratory function. Discussion about fitness for pregnancy should take place between medical staff and the couple planning pregnancy, and the partner of the woman with CF should have their carrier status checked. Unfortunately the majority of CF pregnancies are unplanned and those patients with severe disease will suffer greater morbidity during pregnancy.[12] Sadly, as disease severity progresses, it may be difficult for the young mother to look after both herself and a young child. With a mean survival of adults into the third decade of life, the majority of children born to CF mothers will be motherless by the time the child reaches adolescence.

Self-care, education and compliance

Successfully managing the daily complex routine self-care required of a young CF adult (in addition to working) would be difficult for a healthy adult. Daily care for a CF patient may comprise physiotherapy, nebulisation of bronchodilators and antibiotics, exercise and the taking of considerable amounts of oral medication. There may be difficulties instituting and maintaining preventative care in relatively healthy patients when they do not immediately feel the benefit. As disease severity progresses, further medical interventions are necessary, requiring additional self-care. The commonest of these is regular courses of intravenous antibiotics. A large number of patients can do this successfully at home but will need education and support

The onset of diabetes increases as patients grow older.[13] In the Manchester unit 25% of CF patients are insulin-dependent diabetics. Education to ensure good diabetic control is important.

Box 6.5 Information and protocols for CF patients attending a unit

- a brochure providing information about the unit and available services

- information about allowances

- protocols for using intravenous antibiotics at home, self-care of diabetes, gastrostomy feeding, nebuliser care and exercise programmes

---

Poor control is associated with weight loss, pulmonary deterioration and, possibly, decreased survival.[14] The institution of gastrostomy feeding and non-invasive ventilation in association with preterminal disease create additional burdens with which the patient may have difficulty coping.

It is important that a CF unit provides continuing information and education to CF patients. This can obviously be provided on the basis of one-to-one interviews and a list of publications of specific interest to CF adults is produced by the national bodies (eg, Cystic Fibrosis Research Trust, Alexandra House, 5 Blyth Road, Bromley, Kent BR1 3RJ, UK). On a unit, it is helpful for the patients to have clearly written patient information booklets and defined treatment protocols for managing their self-care (box 6.5). Staff can use these protocols to teach patients and subsequently patient knowledge can be reassessed at intervals to audit the effectiveness of the teaching programmes. A great deal of time, care and sympathy should be spent in providing medical care in out-patients and in hospital to patients who eventually may be physically incapable of sufficient self-care. This maxim applies especially to the very breathless patient.

It is essential that every young adolescent undertakes responsibility for self-care following transfer to an adult CF unit. Compliance may be treatment-specific, being worse for physiotherapy and better for exercise.[15] The former is repetitive and onerous and the latter allows social integration. Compliance is influenced neither by disease severity nor intelligence of the patient. It is better when patients can gain obvious benefits, such as taking their pancreatic supplements in order to avoid the social embarrassment of foul-smelling stools. The ability of physicians to predict compliance accurately does not infer that they can change it. Treatment may need to be tailored to fit a patient's lifestyle, and understanding some of the complex reasons for poor patient compliance may improve the situation. Non-compliance has been classified into three categories by one group, a) inadequate knowledge, b) psychosocial resistance, and c) educated non-adherence.[16]

Using coercion as a method of improving compliance will fail and Lask suggested five main principles[17] for communicating and improving compliance with young CF adults (box 6.6).

Box 6.6 Managing compliance: approaches

- empathy; warm, pragmatic, non-judgemental approach; acknowledge limits to total compliance
- enthusiasm; communicate confidence and provide inspiration
- exploration; spend time understanding the patient's reasons for poor compliance (may be due to poor information, pressure on time, chaotic lifestyle, etc)
- education; may not improve compliance but if information is inadequate compliance will not improve
- expression of emotion; allow the patient to express feelings which might be a mixture of fear, anger, resentment, depression, etc.

Transplantation

Mortality for CF can be predicted on the basis of deterioration in pulmonary function. Patients with an FEV_1 of less than 30% predicted have a 50% chance of dying within two years.[18] At this point in time, consideration should be given for referral for transplantation assessment. This approach may acutely disrupt the CF patient's well-adjusted defences and sense of well being. Patients with severe disease sometimes have no perception of how ill they have become. Communicating objective information of impending mortality requires skill and tact. It may be the first time that patients and their families have faced the terminal nature of CF. It may take several interviews involving close partners to communicate satisfactorily the need for a transplant. Separate input may be required from social workers and doctors. The patient may object to the need for transplantation but, paradoxically with deteriorating health and quality of life, may become demanding for it to occur. With the death of the patient, failing to have got a transplant may leave considerable bitterness and prolonged grieving in the family of the deceased. Occasionally a patient will refuse transplantation which can cause considerable disharmony within the family.

There is the associated paradox that transplantation is both a life-saving and life-threatening operation. There will be patient awareness on a CF unit, that organ transplants in their peers will have been both successful and unsuccessful. A large number of patients have grown up together and death in this manner of a CF friend can cause emotional havoc. Listing for transplantation requires further intensification of self-care. The majority of patients at the Manchester unit have a feeding gastrostomy inserted at time of listing. If respiratory failure with carbon dioxide retention is developing then non-invasive nocturnal ventilation is instituted.

The future

Young people with CF are extremely knowledgeable. They keep up to date with medical advances via the media and their own publications. The former often indulge in hype with regard to scientific breakthroughs, which are heralded as imminent cures. Although the discovery of the gene, the cloning of the CF mouse, and the correction of the basic defect in nasal epithelium are momentus scientific breakthroughs, their transformation into curative therapy may be a decade away. The optimism of patients must be sustained but moderated. Carers of CF patients need to keep up-to-date with current medical and scientific advances.

Improving communication and education, and judging effectiveness

The relationship of the doctor with young adults with CF is different from most doctor/patient relationships. It commences in adolescence between the ages 16-18 and continues over a decade until transplantation or death. During this association, there will be many medical and personal vicissitudes. One of the most important reasons for failure of interaction between carer and patient is poor communication.[19] Improving communications can be considered both from the carers' and patients' perspective.

Carers' perspective

It is essential that the doctor has adequate knowledge of CF.[20] CF is the commonest inherited genetic disease with 6000 patients in the UK. It is essential that medical students and doctors receive some education in this speciality during their training. Information can be provided by the carers to patients, usually at repeated clinical interviews, but much self-care is complex and should be supported with simple written protocols for patients to use at home. Information is not always received correctly and often may be misinterpreted.

What is the best approach to young people with CF? Every patient is different. Often they will require privacy in their discussions without the presence of parents or partners if the subject matter is delicate. Sometimes, it may be important, with the patient's permission, to interview relatives separately so that all the issues are clearly understood. It is important for the carer to be tolerant and have empathy with the patient. It is important to maintain a professional approach but on occasions this may be tested to the limits by rudeness or bad behaviour on the part of the patient. Sometimes the patients will simply follow their own course of action.

Patient's perspective

CF adults are extremely well informed.[21] They publish their own journal containing medical and personal articles, and a handbook of practical information with regard to allowances, housing, insurance, travel, etc. However, they are always seeking more information.[22] The effectiveness of communication from the patient's view will depend upon the approach of the doctor. If the maxims mentioned above are followed then the relationship will prosper. Indifference, disinterest and a superior approach will doom any communication.

Although the discussion has emphasised the importance of

communicating with young adults with CF at various levels, there have been very few studies assessing effectiveness. A recent paper has studied the ability of young CF adults to manage their own disease, which involved self-monitoring and communicating symptoms and disease progress.[23] An important component of this study involved communicating with the CF team. Measuring the efficacy of patients' self-care may reflect the ability of the carers to communicate and educate.

Conclusion

Caring and communicating with young adults with CF is difficult and testing. They are a cross-section of the population who also have CF and communicating about the many difficult issues of the disease may not be the same for each individual. However, the essential component of the doctor/patient relationship is to establish mutual trust. From this firm base everything will be much easier.

I am grateful to Mary Dodd, Shauna Smith and Joan Fitzjohn for the constructive comments in the preparation of this chapter.

1 Dodge JA, Morison S, Lewis PA, et al. Cystic fibrosis in the United Kingdom, 1968-1988: incidence, population and survival. *Paediatr Perinat Epidemiol* 1993;7:157-66.

2 Elborn JS, Shale DJ, Britton JR. Cystic fibrosis: current survival and population estimates to the year 2000. *Thorax* 1991;46:881-5.

3 Walters S, Britton J, Hodson ME. Demographic and social characteristics of adults with cystic fibrosis in the United Kingdom. *BMJ* 1993;306:549-52.

4 Shepherd SL, Harwood IR, Granger LE, et al. A comparative study of the psychosocial assets of adults with cystic fibrosis and their healthy peers. *Chest* 1990;97:1310-6.

5 Blair C, Cull A, Freeman CP. Psychosocial functioning of young adults with cystic fibrosis and their families. *Thorax* 1994; 49: 798-802.

6 Strauss DG, Wellisch DK. Psychosocial adaptations in older cystic fibrosis patients. *J Chronic Dis* 1981;34:141-6.

7 Abbott J, Dodd M, Webb AK. Different perceptions of disease severity and self care between patients with cystic fibrosis, their close companions and physician. *Thorax* 1995;50:794-6.

8 Royal College of Physicians. *Cystic fibrosis adults; recommendations for care in the United Kingdom*. London: Royal College of Physicians, 1990.

9 British Paediatric Association Working Party on Cystic Fibrosis. Cystic Fibrosis in the United Kingdom 1977-1985: an improving picture. *BMJ* 1988;297:1599-603.

10 Walters S, Britton J, Hodson ME. Hospital care for adults with cystic fibrosis: an overview and comparison between specialist cystic fibrosis clinics and general clinics using a patient questionnaire. *Thorax* 1994;49:300-6.

11 Nielsen OH, Schiotz PO. Cystic fibrosis in Denmark in the period 1945-1981: evaluation of centralised treatment. *Acta Paediatr Scand* 1982;**301** (suppl);107-19.

12 Edenborough FP, Stableforth DE, Webb AK, MacKenzie WE, Smith DL. Outcome of pregnancy in cystic fibrosis. *Thorax* 1995;**50**:170-4.

13 Lanng S, Thorsteinsson B, Erichsen G, *et al*. Glucose tolerance in cystic fibrosis. *Arch Dis Child* 1991;**66**:612-6.

14 Finkelstein SM, Wielinski CL, Elliot GR, *et al*. Diabetes mellitus associated with cystic fibrosis. *J Pediatr* 1988;**112**:373-7.

15 Abbott J, Dodd M, Bilton D, Webb AK. Treatment compliance in adults with cystic fibrosis. *Thorax* 1994;**49**:115-20.

16 Koocher G, McGrath M. Gudas L. Typologies of nonadherence in cystic fibrosis. *Dev Behav Paediatr* 1990;**11**:353-8.

17 Lask B. Non-adherence to treatment in cystic fibrosis. *J R Soc Med* 1994;**87**:25-7.

18 Kerem E, Reisman J, Corey M, Canny GJ, Levison H. Prediction of mortality in patients with cystic fibrosis. *N Engl J Med* 1992;**362**:1187-91.

19 Korsch BM, Negrete VF. Doctor-patient communication. *Sci Am* 1972;**227**:66-72.

20 Webb AK, David TJ. Clinical management of children and adults with cystic fibrosis: education and debate. *BMJ* 1994;**308**:459-62.

21 Nolan T, Desmond K, Herlich R, Hardy S. Knowledge of cystic fibrosis in patients and their parents. *Pediatrics* 1986;**77**:229-35.

22 Hames A, Beesley J, Nelson R. Cystic fibrosis: what do patients know, and what else would they like to know. *Respir Med* 1991;**85**:389-92.

23 Bartholomew LK, Parcel GS, Swank PR, Czywski DI. Measuring self-efficacy expectations for the self management of cystic fibrosis. *Chest* 1993;**103**:1524-30.

7 Counselling for an HIV test

SHEILA MOSS, OLWEN E WILLIAMS,
CHARLES RK HIND

We are now fifteen years into the AIDS epidemic and public attitudes towards HIV, AIDS and HIV antibody testing have changed. The United Kingdom Department of Health no longer expects specialist counsellors to have the sole remit for pre-test discussion but anticipate that discussion about HIV and HIV testing should be part of mainstream clinical care.[1] The aim of this chapter is to give a practical guide to all doctors who may need to counsel and test their patients for the presence of HIV antibodies (box 7.1). Its aims are to answer the questions: why? when? how? where? and who?[2] Counselling for an HIV test is not a form of psychotherapy and should really be referred to as "pre-test discussion". It is not a lengthy procedure despite the fact that large books written on the subject have added to its mystique and user unfriendliness. The skills required are no different from those necessary in any clinical situation. Namely, awareness, sensitivity and good communication.

Box 7.1 Aims of counselling before an HIV antibody test

- to provide information on the technical aspects of screening
- to provide information on the possible implications of being diagnosed positive or negative (eg, medical, social and legal)
- to educate on the risks of transmission, and discuss behaviour that might reduce these risks

---

Doctors are often too embarrassed to ask patients about HIV related issues so information may not be shared. Patients may be concerned that the illness may be HIV related and be afraid to ask. They may have already been HIV tested or recently donated blood in which case they will know their HIV status but consider it inappropriate to tell the doctor.

Why test?

Patients sometimes believe that as long as they are not placing anyone else at risk, a knowledge of their own HIV status is unnecessary. This is no longer the case. Time and many clinical trials have shown improved long-term outcome in those HIV positive patients who are aware of their infection, and who are treated prophylactically at appropriate stages of their illness against opportunistic infections.[3] Treatment with antiretroviral agents has also improved outcome[4] and may reduce the rate of vertical transmission from mother to child. The introduction of antenatal HIV screening is being strongly driven by the Department of Health in the UK.[6] Detailed discussion about sexual practices and lifestyle may also allow for behaviour modification, and therefore a reduction of overall risk to the patient and partner.

These and other issues, for which guidelines have been published by the World Health Organization[7] form the basis of pre-test discussion. In most instances "informed consent" is being sought. This involves giving the patient information about the nature of the tests and the medical, social, and legal implications of the result. Clearly, the information given must be tailored to the individual's needs. It is assumed that the patient has the capacity to understand the information provided, in order to assess the risks and benefits of testing.

HIV testing scenarios

The individual may present actively seeking HIV testing for the first time or for a repeat test. However, it may be that HIV is part of the differential diagnosis and the individual is unaware that their symptoms may be related to the virus.

HIV testing may be part of a wider screening procedure such as the following three scenarios:

● antenatal care

- blood donation
- a health check for insurance purposes or travel or immigration

Basic information procedures to follow in each scenario can be tailored to suit the particular setting in which it is conducted.

Out-patient testing

HIV pre-test discussion may arise in the out-patient setting as part of an investigation of an illness or at the patient's request. Some individuals still believe that "having a blood test" for whatever reason means they have been tested for HIV and this must be clarified. As part of the introduction, you should ensure that the individual is aware of the nature of the HIV test, the difference between HIV and AIDS, the modes of transmission, and the methods which can reduce the risk of transmission which the individual currently uses and should be encouraged to use. Therefore, it is important that at this point a detailed history of sexual activities, drug use, past infections, foreign travel, exposure to high risk activity and any occupational risk be evaluated as this will give the doctor a clear understanding of the likelihood of infection. The discussion involves assessing the patient's understanding of risk and discussion of high risk behaviour. It also reassures the patient that everyday social and domestic activities are safe. Underlying this process are the dual aims of prevention and support. The patient should be assured of continued medical care no matter what the result is.

It is important that the timing of the test does not fall within the three month "window period". This should be explained and the test repeated if that individual is within the "window period" to ensure a reliable result. Consensus of opinion is that a single test at three months will diagnose the majority.[8]

Advantages and disadvantages of testing should be discussed. It is also important at this point to discuss with the patient how he or she would cope should the test result be positive as this may help minimise adverse psychological consequences.[9] It also allows the health care worker to inform the patient of the social and psychological support available.

In some areas of the US written consent has been sought. In the UK written consent is only requested by blood donors and purchasers of life assurance, neither of whom may receive formal HIV pre-test discussion. In addition, those who require tests to travel or work abroad, depending on which setting they present, should ideally receive pre-test discussion although this is not always the case.

Post test information involves a discussion of both the result and if positive with whom the patient wishes to share the information, for example, partner, doctor, dentist. It also allows information regarding safer sex, injecting practices, treatment options and follow up to be discussed if appropriate. In the case of a negative HIV test, the opportunity for reasserting safer sexual or injecting practices is important.

These recommendations for HIV pre-test information are based on out-patient settings consisting of genitourinary medicine clinics and same day testing services where the worried but otherwise well person requests testing. It is also important that written material is available as an individual may choose to defer testing until they have contemplated the issues further.

In-patient testing

In clinical practice, doctors are most likely to discuss HIV testing with a seriously ill patient who is investigating for one more condition, as listed in box 7.2. It is important that a rapid diagnosis is reached and it may be inappropriate to delay testing. It is imperative that the doctor feels comfortable in performing the pre-test discussion rather than asking another member of staff to see

---

Box 7.2 Physical conditions which may indicate underlying HIV infection

- tuberculosis
- extensive fungal infection (eg, candidiasis)
- extensive herpes zoster
- persistent lymphadenopathy
- persistent diarrhoea
- unexplained weight loss
- oral hairy leucoplakia
- kaposi's sarcoma
- pyrexia of unknown origin (PUO)
- lymphopenia
- thrombocytopenia
- severe community acquired pneumonia

---

the patient in order to discuss HIV testing. This may delay the process and increase the patient's sense of isolation and guilt and fear. However, in some instances, it may be more appropriate for the patient to be directed to a department of genitourinary medicine where screening for other sexually transmitted infections, hepatitis B and syphilis may also be carried out.

When HIV testing a seriously ill patient in order to make a diagnosis, a doctor is acting in the patient's best interests. Informed consent should normally be obtained, however, there area few exceptions; for instance, for a life saving procedure when the patient is unconscious and cannot indicate his or her wishes; where a minor is a ward of court and the court decides this specific treatment is in the child's best interests; or for the treatment of a physical disorder when a patient is incapable of giving consent by reason of a mental disorder and the treatment is in the patient's best interests (box 7.3).

Box 7.3 Examination or treatment without the patient's consent

The following are examples of occasions when examination or treatment may proceed without obtaining the patient's consent:

- for life saving procedures where the patient is unconscious and cannot indicate his or her wishes
- in certain cases where a minor is a ward of court and the court decides that a specific treatment is in the child's best interests
- treatment for a physical disorder where the patient is incapable of giving consent by reason of mental disorder, and the treatment is in the patient's best interests

---

In contrast to the out-patient scenario there is unlikely to be a quiet setting, and it is therefore important, if possible, to be able to talk to the patient in a quiet area of the ward in absolute privacy. Allow up to 15 uninterrupted minutes for the process. A discussion of diagnostic possibilities and the results of investigations to date may be a helpful introduction to the pre-test discussion. If there is clinical or laboratory evidence of HIV, this should be disclosed. It may be useful to ask if the patient has any thoughts as to why this might be. Enquiring about any risk factors in an indirect way is also important, for instance, by asking about marital status, sexual partners, any past history of sexually transmitted infections. Past history of blood transfusion, travel abroad, glandular fever like illness, and drug use should be taken. Also ask the patient about the possibility of any previous tests. As individuals are tested when they donate blood, it is important to ask if they have ever been a blood donor. This also might have implications if they gave blood during the "window period". If their immediate management might be changed through being HIV positive, explain this to them. Ask them if they would be willing to have an HIV test performed. It is appropriate to indicate how long the test will take and who will give the result. Explain that if the test is positive, a confirmatory test will be required on another blood sample. Further discussion regarding partners, insurance, further information on HIV, can be deferred until another time. A checklist of points to cover may be helpful (box 7.4).

Box 7.4 Pre-test discussion checklist

- introduce yourself and identify your role
- assess risk factors
- explore HIV/AIDS
- explain test procedures (a blood sample; confirmation of a positive result with a second sample)
- discuss possible advantages, including
  - early diagnosis and treatment
  - reassurance, certainty, early treatment
  - better motivation for safer sex, safer drug use
- discuss possible disadvantages, including
  - mortgage and life assurance
  - social relationship prospects
- discuss coping with a negative or positive result; identify personal, social and medical support systems
- discuss how to protect sexual partner(s) in the meantime (safer sex and/or safer drug use)
- if female, discuss pregnancy and fertility
- discuss who to tell and who has been told

Antenatal testing

The potential advantage of early diagnosis of HIV infection is exemplified by the intervention in pregnancy of antiretroviral therapy which reduces the risk of vertical transmission from 25% to 8·3%.[5] Avoidance of breastfeeding in a HIV positive woman has also been shown to reduce the risk to the infant considerably.[10] The unlinked anonymous surveys in England and Wales have demonstrated that in pregnant women a significant number of infections are undiagnosed.[11] Centres with a high prevalence of HIV positive pregnant women should routinely offer HIV testing.[6] Antenatal clinics and midwives[12] are well placed to undertake pre-test discussion and the women need to be informed not only of the advantages and disadvantages of the test in general, but also the benefits of knowing their status during pregnancy and how the outcome can be influenced as such. Written information is also appropriate in this setting as part of the general antenatal information package.

Confidentiality

Confidentiality is a very difficult problem. All medical staff have a legal duty to maintain confidentiality of a patient's personal health information. Many articles on counselling stress how vital it is to ensure the patient's "absolute confidentiality". In reality when an HIV positive patient becomes a hospital in-patient and his or her diagnosis is written in the hospital notes, confidentiality is a relative thing, as it is for all hospital in-patients. Medical notes should, at all times, be "absolutely confidential". However, investigations with the patient's diagnosis and name written on them are sent to other departments or hospitals routinely. Thus, staff not immediately involved in patient care may have access to this information. Patients can be reassured that their HIV results will only be seen for "medical" reasons by doctors and nurses involved in their care. Also information written on forms can be modified so that a diagnosis of HIV is not immediately obvious. Samples must, of course, be labelled "high risk" but phrases such as "low T4 count" or "retroviral illness" may be used. The patient may often be reassured that the front of their notes will not be changed in order to identify infection. Those tested in a department of genitourinary medicine will have additional confidentiality provided by Section 2 of the NHS Venereal Disease Regulations 1974.

It is important to discuss with the patient who they want to be made aware of their HIV diagnosis, partners, their family doctor, dentist, etc. In general, information is best disclosed on a "need to know basis" only.

Life assurance

Patients often want to discuss the implications of HIV testing for life assurance. There are two ground rules:

● any insurance or endowment policy taken out before 1988 remains valid

● insurance companies currently ask "Have you ever had an HIV antibody test or advice and counselling about AIDS?"[13]

Clearly it is up to the individual to be honest. In order not to discriminate against the socially responsible patient who has had a negative HIV test (who is not necessarily at risk), the Association of British Insurers has recommended that proposers should not be asked about negative HIV tests.[15] Insurers say that they will soon ask the question "Have you ever tested positive for HIV?" This is the question asked in Canada, France and the US, where no significance is attached to a previous negative HIV test.[15] Currently, insurance companies do not consider screening for antenatal purposes, life assurance and travel as being relevant.

Giving the result

Telling patients they are HIV positive is not easy, just like breaking any bad news. It is best done by the doctor who counselled the patient and performed the test. It helps if the patient is aware of when and by whom this result is going to be given and that this information is adhered to. A patient who is prepared for receiving a positive result may still be shocked, angry or go into denial and appear totally unaffected by the result. As with the pre-test discussion, it is important to give the result in a setting where there will be no interruptions, and sometimes it is appropriate to negotiate a third party to be present when the result is given. Always have a plan of action on giving a result; what the next step is going to be; who will be looking after the individual; which further tests need to be done (for instance, CD4 count to assess level of immunosuppression), which therapeutic interventions are available; and the use of antiretroviral medication. Also be prepared for such questions as "How long have I been infected?" At this point, the patient may want to discuss who else may have been infected or who he or she may have caught the infection from. You may even be asked to break the bad news to the patient's sexual partner. It is also important to have written information about HIV and AIDS available and also a list of useful telephone numbers such as voluntary agencies, support groups and social work facilities. Over this period, the individual will need a lot of support from medical and nursing staff.

Ethical considerations

In November 1995, the General Medical Council released a series of booklets concerning the duties of a doctor. One of the four booklets was entitled *HIV and AIDS, the ethical considerations*. It covers aspects of the doctor–patient relationship, a doctor's duties towards patients, duties of doctors infected with the virus, consent to HIV testing, confidentiality, informing other healthcare professionals and informing the patient's spouse and sexual partner. This booklet is essential reading for all doctors, regardless of their speciality, and has been distributed to all doctors registered with the GMC.

Conclusion

In conclusion, by discussing HIV-related issues routinely with the patients, doctors will feel more comfortable about dealing with them. Doctors should not look upon HIV testing as a particular problem. It is simply yet another challenge to their skills and abilities to communicate with their patients and improve the quality of their care.

1   Department of Health. *Guidelines for pre-test discussion on HIV testing.* PL/CMO/96. London: Department of Health, 1996.
2   Kipling R. *The Elephant's Child.*
3   Peters BS, Coleman D, Becks EJ, *et al.* Changing disease patterns in AIDS. *BMJ* 1991;**302**:726-31.
4   Fishel MA, Richman DD, Grieco MH, *et al.* The efficacy of azidothymidine in the treatment of patients with AIDS and AIDS related complex; an open uncontrolled treatment study. *N Engl J Med* 1987;**317**:185-91.
5   Conner EM, Sperling RS, Gelber R, *et al.* Reduction of maternal-infant transmission of human immunodeficiency virus Type I with zidovudine treatment. *N Engl J Med* 1994;**331**:1173-80.
6   Department of Health. Department of Health guidance PL/CO/(92)5, appendix 2. *Guidelines for offering voluntary named HIV antibody testing to women receiving antenatal care.* London: Department of Health, 1992.
7   World Health Organization. *Guidelines for counselling about HIV infection and disease.* Geneva: WHO, 1990.

8   The British Co-operative Clinical Group; When to perform the final HIV antibody test following possible exposure. *Int J STD AIDS* 1995;6:332-5.

9   Miller R, Bor R. *AIDS: a guide to clinical counselling.* London: Science Press, 1988.

10 Dunn DT, Newell ML, Ades AE, Peckham CS. Risk of human immuno deficiency virus Type I transmission through breastfeeding. *Lancet* 1992;340:585-8.

11 Department of Health, Public Health Service, Institute of Child Health. Unlinked Anonymous HIV Surveys Steering Group. Unlinked anonymous HIV seroprevalence monitoring programme in England and Wales; data to the end of 1995. London: December, 1996.

12 Chryslie IL, Wolfe CDA, *et al.* Voluntary named testing for HIV in a community based antenatal clinic: pilot study. *BMJ* 1995;311:928-31.

13 Barton SE, Roth P. Life assurance and HIV antibody testing. *BMJ* 1992;305:902-3.

14 Byrne L. Insurers relax questions on HIV. *BMJ* 1994; 309: 359.

15 Reynolds MA, Barton SE, Singh S, *et al.* HIV and insurance commentary. *Int J STD AIDS* 1994;5:322-6.

8 A patient with multiple sclerosis

HELEN L FORD, MICHAEL H JOHNSON

Making the diagnosis of multiple sclerosis

Multiple sclerosis is probably one of the most feared diseases to affect young and middle aged adults. Making and communicating the diagnosis is, therefore, crucially important.

The historical name for the disease, "disseminated sclerosis" reminded us that in order to make the diagnosis, there had to be evidence of lesions occurring in different parts of the nervous system at different points in the history. By definition, therefore, the diagnosis can hardly ever be made at the time when the first symptoms occur. There are exceptions to this general rule. A young woman with a definite episode of optic neuritis in the past, who now has an internuclear ophthalmoplegia, a pale optic disc with a relative afferent pupillary defect, bladder problems and extensor plantar responses can be confidently told the diagnosis. Another young woman with a sensory disturbance starting in her feet and spreading up to the waist, lasting two to three weeks before starting to recede, has very probably got multiple sclerosis but does not fulfill the diagnostic criteria and may need to be investigated to exclude another spinal cord lesion.

An experienced doctor may suspect multiple sclerosis at the first visit in many patients with an episode of neurological disturbance, but it may take some years, if and when a second episode occurs, before the diagnostic criteria are fulfilled and the patient can be confidently told what is wrong. The patient may then complain of having been kept in the dark all the time. Should the doctor have voiced a suspicion of a frightening disease at the first stage, knowing that some patients would not go on to get the disease-defining second episode? If you ask patients later, many express bitterness that the diagnosis was not discussed, but there are one or two who report that they are glad that the suspicion of the disease was not voiced.

Do investigations help?

Multiple sclerosis is diagnosed on clinical grounds and it is folly to rely entirely on investigation results. The value of investigations is probably exaggerated and a logical approach is needed. If the patient has a relapsing and remitting condition which could result from a single lesion of the central nervous system (CNS), you need to do a test which demonstrates clinically silent lesions elsewhere. There is not a lot of point in doing visual evoked potentials in someone with optic neuritis but they can be useful in someone with a brainstem or cervical cord syndrome. Magnetic resonance imaging (MRI) can show multiple lesions characteristic of multiple sclerosis which will help to confirm the diagnosis in a young person with purely spinal cord symptoms and signs. The analysis of cerebrospinal fluid (CSF) is probably more useful, and just as sensitive, in someone with symptoms indicating disseminated lesions but with few or no signs. The table demonstrates the influence of positive MRI and/or positive oligoclonal bands on the classification of multiple sclerosis according to the Poser criteria.[1] The importance of historical and clinical examination findings in classification is evident. A very useful discipline is to ask yourself why you are doing the test and what you will tell the patient if it is *(a)* positive, *(b)* negative, or *(c)* inconclusive.

What should the patient be told?

Possible diagnosis

Patients these days are increasingly likely to have suspected the diagnosis but they may not express their fear explicitly. If you are sure that multiple sclerosis is very unlikely, it may be useful to tell the patient that you don't think they have a serious condition such as multiple sclerosis or Parkinson's disease. If you think they might have multiple sclerosis, give the patient every opportunity to voice their fears. Ask them if they have any thoughts about what might

Table 8.1 The influence of positive MRI and/or positive oligoclonal bands in the CSF on the Poser diagnostic classification of multiple sclerosis.

History (no. of attacks)	Clinical evidence	MRI /oligoclonal bands	Poser class
2	2 lesions	Clinical diagnosis	Clinically definite multiple sclerosis
2	1 lesion	+ MRI	Clinically definite multiple sclerosis
		– MRI	Clinically probable multiple sclerosis
2	1 lesion	+ oligoclonal bands	Laboratory supported definite multiple sclerosis
		– oligoclonal bands	Clinically probable multiple sclerosis
1	1 lesion	+ MRI* + oligoclonal bands	Laboratory supported definite multiple sclerosis
1	1 lesion	+ MRI* – oligoclonal bands	Clinically probable multiple sclerosis
1	1 lesion	– MRI + oligoclonal bands	Not diagnostic
1	1 lesion	– MRI – oligoclonal bands	Not diagnostic

*ie, new lesions developing on follow-up MRI after 1 month or more. Single MRI not diagnostic as no "dissemination in time".

be wrong. Ask if any particular condition worries them. Once they say the dreaded words, it is then much easier to explain whether it is likely or unlikely and to explain what steps may need to be taken to find out. Although most people asked in the street "Would you wish to be informed if you had multiple sclerosis?" would naturally say "Yes", when it comes to it, there are definite disadvantages to being told. First of all, it may be difficult to get life insurance or promotion at work, the threat of a disabling condition may alter life plans inappropriately, and strains between partners may be introduced. It is as well to point out these potential problems before going ahead with investigations which may not be clinically necessary.

Box 8.1 Telling your patient he or she has multiple sclerosis: how not to do it

A young woman is referred to a neurologist complaining of a numb leg. She goes with her husband for the initial consultation where they are reassured that no serious disease seems to be present. However, the doctor suggests that since they have private medical insurance, it wouldn't hurt to ask for an MRI which would show such things as a thoracic disc.

Two weeks later, the patient, who has by now recovered, goes back on her own to get the result and is told that the scan showed multiple sclerosis. She doesn't recall what was said after that, but had to drive home on her own, collect the children from school, and wait to tell her husband when he comes home. It's a day she is unlikely to forget.

If the patient does not express any concerns about the possibility of having multiple sclerosis, you are in much greater difficulty. You can investigate the current symptoms sufficiently to exclude another treatable condition, but if it becomes clear that multiple sclerosis is likely you have to allow time for adequate discussion and sooner or later the diagnosis must be discussed.

Definite diagnosis

Most people with multiple sclerosis report dissatisfaction with the way in which they were told they had the disease (see boxes 8.1-8.3). They also report anger over the delay in the prompt provision of a diagnosis. In a retrospective survey in Southampton,[2]

Box 8.2 Telling your patient he or she has multiple sclerosis: how not to do it

A middle aged man develops double vision and is found by an opthalmologist to have a sixth nerve palsy. After four weeks, it seems not to be improving and the ophthalmologist requests a CT brain scan. The radiology department notice that he is also on their waiting list for an MRI of his lumbar spine where he has some inflammatory problem. They decide to kill two birds with one scan and arrange a brain MRI on the same day. The ophthalmologist reviews the patient, whose double vision has now completely recovered, and reads out the report of the scan which "diagnoses" multiple sclerosis. The patient now has difficulty getting a mortgage for his business premises even though, three years later, the clinical diagnosis of multiple sclerosis has not been established and he may have some other connective tissue/inflammatory disorder.

Box 8.3 Telling your patient he or she has multiple sclerosis: how not to do it

A young woman with vague neurological symptoms is concerned that she may have multiple sclerosis. The neurologist finds nothing definite but requests investigations. The evoked potentials are suspicious and the neurologist tells her that she probably has multiple sclerosis. The next time she comes to the clinic, a different doctor re-examines her and says she probably doesn't have multiple sclerosis. The CSF and MRI are normal, but she still has symptoms and some doctors tell her it is multiple sclerosis while others say it isn't.

---

approximately 60% of the population of people with multiple sclerosis felt that they were not given enough information at the time of diagnosis.

Doctors often feel that the diagnosis of multiple sclerosis should be delayed as long as possible to reduce the emotional burden on the patient. However a recent prospective study of people with suspected multiple sclerosis[3] provides no support for this practice. The health perceptions of people with suspected multiple sclerosis were studied over a six month period during which time they underwent a diagnostic "workup". In those with a definitive diagnosis there was less overall anxiety and less distress about physical symptoms. A further component of the study was to examine the value of diagnostic information to people with suspected multiple sclerosis.[4] Those patients with a definitive diagnosis reported an increased sense of wellbeing and a slight improvement in quality of life after diagnosis. However those patients in whom no definitive diagnosis emerged tended to be more anxious rather than reassured by the negative results.

Positive aspects of diagnosis

People with suspected multiple sclerosis have usually had neurological symptoms for some time before presentation to a neurologist. A diagnosis of multiple sclerosis may be reassuring to people fearing they have a brain tumour or that their symptoms are due to mental illness. Patients are thought generally to benefit from earlier diagnosis.[5]

The development of new treatments for multiple sclerosis such as interferon beta-1b, interferon beta-1a and copolymer-1 has important implications for early diagnosis as these drugs seem to be most beneficial, on present evidence, at an early stage of the disease.[6,7]

Guidelines for imparting the diagnosis[8]

The British Society of Rehabilitation Medicine with the support of the Multiple Sclerosis Society of Great Britain and Northern Ireland published guidelines for imparting the diagnosis of multiple sclerosis in April 1993 (see boxes 8.4 and 8.5). These guidelines were based on information from retrospective surveys of people with multiple sclerosis.

Box 8.4 What do people with multiple sclerosis want to know?

- general information
- what symptoms might be expected? A working prognosis
- future disability
  - Will I end up in a wheelchair?
  - Will multiple sclerosis affect my mind?
  - Will I be able to work?
  - Will I die of it?
- is there any treatment?
- what causes multiple sclerosis?
- will it affect my children? Implications for future pregnancy
- self-help measures: suitable activities, exercise, diet
- contact groups: Multiple Sclerosis Society

Box 8.5 Guidelines for imparting the diagnosis of multiple sclerosis

- people with multiple sclerosis expect a clear explanation for their symptoms which in the vast majority of cases involves communicating the specific diagnosis to the patient
- many people prefer a relative or friend to be with them
- the doctor giving the diagnosis must have adequate knowledge of the disease and adequate time
- it is thought to be helpful for the doctor to give a "working prognosis" for the next 12 months
- a follow-up appointment to see the doctor who has discussed the diagnosis should be offered
- information should be given about the local Multiple Sclerosis Society supplemented by appropriate written information about the disease

---

Don't forget that others also "suffer" from the diagnosis; ask the patient what he or she wants to tell the family. Children in particular may have unwarranted fears about the condition.

It may be useful if a specialist nurse is able to talk to the patient and provide valuable counselling without the time constraints of an outpatient clinic. Written information or specialist video films can be of great benefit for patients to refer to at home. It is essential that an early follow-up appointment is made so that the patient has a chance to ask questions in a calmer state of mind.

The Multiple Sclerosis Society and other self help groups can provide support and information, but this should not be rushed. Well meaning relatives or friends or professionals may overload the patient with advice and information, and a visit to a local branch of the Multiple Sclerosis Society may be a depressing experience for a newly diagnosed patient.

Counselling can be helpful but it is not a simple solution. Somebody with training and experience in communicating "bad news" may be able to help the patient go through processes akin to a bereavement reaction. Even a very experienced neurologist cannot predict the course of severity of a patient's disease and investigations are of very little help in predicting the future course of the disease.

What information can we give?

Multiple sclerosis is a chronic neurological disorder affecting one person per thousand of the UK population. The cause is unknown. At present there is no medical cure, although there are treatments which can help many of the symptoms.

Course of multiple sclerosis

The course of multiple sclerosis is different in each individual and can be difficult to predict. Initially the disease may be relapsing and remitting with full recovery between relapses. The length of relapse varies greatly between 24 hours and 12 months.[9] The annual relapse rate varies widely in different studies from 0·1 to 1·15 relapses per year.[10] Relapse is more common in the first five years after onset and particularly in the first year.

The disease may become progressive at any time after the onset. Secondary progression occurs in about 40% of patients by 10 years after onset and in 60% by 15 years. Progression is not, however, inevitable. McAlpine states that in any series of patients seen soon after onset 33% will be benign at 10 years, 25% at 15 years and 20% at 20 years.[10] Primary progression from the onset of the disease seems to occur in 10-20% of cases. There is a clear relationship between progressive disease and late age of onset.

Employment

In the first five years from onset different authors have found that up to 50% of patients were in full work and up to 70% were capable of some work. By 15 years between 10-25% were in full work with up to 40% of long term survivors capable of some useful activity. Spastic paresis of the legs is the major cause of the loss of ability to work. Incoordination, sphincter disturbance and fatigue are also significant factors with many patients having more than one disability. More patients could work if there were better access to the workplace or if they could work from home.

Life expectancy

The degree of disability at any given time is the strongest indicator of life expectancy. The cause of death is not usually a direct effect of multiple sclerosis but results from infective complications or from unrelated disease. Life expectancy for people with multiple sclerosis has been found to be only about 6 to 7 years less than the insured population without multiple sclerosis from the ages 20 to 50 and this difference is even less after age 50.[11] Many individuals live a normal lifespan.

Aetiology

The cause or causes of multiple sclerosis are not known. There is evidence that an environmental factor may play a role and that some individuals are more susceptible to this factor and thus more likely to develop the disease. Whether a person will or will not develop multiple sclerosis is thought to have been determined by the age of approximately 15 years.

Pregnancy

There is a slightly increased risk of relapse in some women during the first three months after they have given birth. However the overall course of the disease is not altered by pregnancy. Fertility is not reduced and there is no increased risk of spontaneous abortion or stillbirth. There are no specific complications of labour and no contraindications to breast feeding.

Genetics

Multiple sclerosis does occur more commonly in relatives of affected patients than in the rest of the population. Usually only two individuals are affected and the commonest relationship is sibship. The risk of a child being affected is less and is thought to be 1-4%.

Self help measures

There is no scientific evidence at present that specific diets alter the course of the disease. The practical results of therapeutic trials involving dietary supplementation with polyunsaturated fatty acids have been disappointing. However, many patients are keen to do something positive themselves and do adapt their diets to include more liquid vegetable fats and unsaturated margarine.

There may be a temporary aggravation of induction of symptoms of multiple sclerosis with exertion. However there is little to suggest that unaccustomed exertion may induce relapse. Common advice is to avoid excessive fatigue but otherwise to continue normal activities.

1   Poser CM, Paty DW, Scheinberg L, *et al.* New diagnostic criteria for multiple sclerosis: guidelines for research protocols. *Ann Neurol* 1983;**13**:227-31.

2   McLellan DL, Martin JR, Roberts MHW, Spackman A, McIntosh-Michaelis S, Nichols S. Multiple sclerosis in the Southampton District. University of Southampton: Rehabilitation Research Unit and Department of Sociology and Social Policy, 1989.

3   O'Connor P, Detsky AS, Tansey C, Kucharczyk W. Effect of diagnostic testing for multiple sclerosis on patient health perceptions. *Arch Neurol* 1994;**51**:46-51.

4   Mushlin AI, Mooney C, Grow V, Phelps CE. The value of diagnostic information to patients with suspected MS. *Arch Neurol* 1994;**51**:67-72.

5   Elian M, Dean G. To tell or not to tell the diagnosis of multiple sclerosis. *Lancet* 1985;**2**:27-8.

6   IFNB Multiple Sclerosis Study Group. Interferon beta-1b is effective in relapsing-remitting multiple sclerosis. I. Clinical results of a multicenter, randomized, controlled trial. *Neurology* 1993;**43**:655-61.

7   McDonald WI. New treatments for multiple sclerosis. *BMJ* 1995:**310**:345-6.

8   Multiple sclerosis. A working party report of the British Society of Rehabilitation Medicine. April, 1993.

9   McAlpine D, Compston ND. Some aspects of the natural history of disseminated sclerosis. *Q J Med* 1952;**21**:135-67.

10 Matthews WB, Compston DAS, Allen IV, Martyn CV (eds). *McAlpine's multiple sclerosis.* 2nd ed. Edinburgh: Churchill Livingstone, 1991.

11 Sadovnick AD, Ebers GC, Wilson RW, Paty DW. Life expectancy in patients attending multiple sclerosis clinics. *Neurology* 1992;**42**:991-4.

9 A patient with cancer

MICHAEL BENNET, DAWN L ALISON

Cancer is a common illness with an overall lifetime incidence of one in three. It causes one in four deaths annually in the UK. Doctors are aware of the many different forms that cancer takes and that it is not inevitably fatal. The lay public, although increasingly well informed by the press and media, still tends to view a diagnosis of cancer as an imminent death sentence. Disclosing to patients that they have cancer is accepted practice now in western cultures and there is evidence in support of frank discussion about diagnosis and treatment details with cancer patients.[1,2]

Breaking bad news is difficult and the way in which someone receives news can leave a lasting impression on them. Patients appreciate it being done in a sensitive way and they, along with their relatives, can harbour long-term resentment if it is done badly. It is essential for doctors to prepare for the reality of breaking bad news and to look at ways of improving their skills (see boxes 9.1 and 9.2). The fact that communication ability is a skill that can be taught and improved has been demonstrated

---

Box 9.1 Breaking bad news

- forms part of clinical practice
- it is a skill that can be taught and improved
- patients and relatives appreciate discussion in a sensitive manner
- the degree to which the news is bad depends on the gap between the patient's perception of the situation and reality

---

> **Box 9.2 Benefits of learning to break bad news in a skilful way**
>
> - enables better psychological adjustment by the patient
> - reduces stress in doctors
> - facilitates open discussion between patients, their relatives and their doctors
> - empowers patients by allowing them a greater say in treatment decisions

previously.[3] An increasing number of medical schools now include communication skills teaching in their curricula and clinicians working closely with cancer patients can benefit from tuition in this area.[4] Interactive teaching methods using videos, role play and discussion work well and there are a range of training resources available.[5-7]

Receiving a diagnosis of cancer will almost inevitably be perceived as bad news. It is important to accept that bad news cannot be turned into good news. Calman suggested that quality of life could be conceptualised as the gap between a person's hopes and expectations and that of the realities of their life.[8] An analogy exists when breaking bad news; the degree of bad news is proportional to the distance between the patient's perception of the situation and reality.[9] The task for the doctor is to ease the patient from their perception of the situation to the reality of that situation. The skill in achieving this lies in controlling the speed of the transition in order that the patient can digest the information at his or her pace (see box 9.3). The larger the "gap", the more difficult this can be. It has been argued that too quick a transition can prevent adaptation and induce denial.[10]

The following outline suggests an approach to discussing a diagnosis of cancer with a patient based on our own experience

> **Box 9.3 Objectives of breaking bad news**
>
> - remember that bad news can never be good news
> - the task is to close the gap between the patient's perception of the situation and the reality of the situation
> - the skill lies in controlling the speed of the transition to fit the patient's pace

and recommendations of others. These steps can be adapted to a variety of clinical situations where bad news is being broken and are not designed solely for discussing the diagnosis of cancer.

Preparation for the interview

Adequate preparation and time are essential for breaking bad news in order to avoid psychological scarring for the patient. If a surgeon attempted a difficult elective operation with inadequate operating time, information, or facilities, a stormy postoperative course with the potential for long-term complications could be expected. There are direct parallels when breaking bad news.

Preparation of the patient can be started at early consultations by anticipating situations that are likely to lead to bad news being given. For example, when investigations are being organised, it is best to be realistic and honest. If a doctor suspects that the tests will confirm a clinical suspicion of malignancy (or even if malignancy is a possible differential diagnosis) it is useful to indicate this to the patient. A phrase such as "I'm worried about serious disease and this test will help to exclude it" conveys this. This can also be a useful time to find out how much of the test results patients want to be told and whether they want to be accompanied by a relative or friend at the next consultation. There is a difficult balance between alarming patients unnecessarily and falsely re-assuring them, but there is no room for platitudes or false reassurances as this could lead to a loss of confidence in the doctor at a later stage.

Beginning the interview

The doctor should avoid being rushed, though this is sometimes difficult to achieve. Reading the medical notes carefully and ensuring that the correct information is present is vital before meeting the patient. If the bad news hinges on the results of recent investigations the doctor should read the written reports personally and have them to hand. Using another person's interpretation of the reports can lead to confusion. Privacy is desirable and a separate room is best. The presence of a nurse who is involved with the patient can provide on-going support for the patient and their relatives after the bad news has been given. If the patient wishes relatives to be present during the discussion they should be given

---

Box 9.4 Preparation for the interview

● make time to do it well
● ensure adequate and correct information
● ensure privacy
● introduce yourself and ascertain how others in the room are related to the patient
● sit down and make eye contact
● if the patient is alone, allow time for the relatives to be there if the patient wants this, where possible

---

the opportunity to arrange this wherever possible (see box 9.4). There have been reports of the benefits of tape recording the bad news consultation and this may be an option in some settings.[11,12]

A brief introduction is helpful especially when the doctor has the unenviable task of breaking bad news to a patient that he or she has not met before. A hand shake followed by "I am Dr Smith, the registrar who works with Dr Jones, the consultant you saw last week" enables the patient to place the doctor in context. Even if the patient and doctor have met before the patient may be too anxious to remember the doctor's name or face. It is important to find out the names and relationships of any other accompanying people who are in the room and to check whether the patient feels it is appropriate to speak freely in front of them. The doctor should sit down near the patient at roughly the same level and make eye contact. It is useful to indicate how much time is available in order to avoid fidgeting, clock-watching, or staring into the notes, which will reduce rapport.

Clarifying the patient's story and coping strategy

The patient's interpretation of the illness should be sought by asking about the symptoms, the results of tests so far and what treatment has been given. Finding out the patient's thoughts and feelings at each stage by using open questions and waiting for an answer facilitates this process. A direct enquiry about the patient's understanding of the situation may be necessary, eg, "What do you understand from all the test results you have had?" The patient may have been falsely re-assured at a previous consultation and this is an opportunity for the doctor to judge the gap between the patient's perception and reality. Conversely, the patient may have been well prepared for the bad news such that their "gap" is small and the task is easier.

After the patient's story has been clarified, the patient should be asked whether a further explanation about the illness or the latest results is needed. It is likely that the answer will be "yes" but occasionally may be "I'd rather not know" in which case the doctor should respect that. Patients should not have information forced on them. The patient's coping strategy can be re-assessed later as it may change throughout the illness or even during the interview.

Breaking the news

If the patient has indicated that he or she wants more information then the doctor can proceed. Explaining slowly using congruent, non-verbal communication and a gentle but solemn voice is best. Giving a warning such as "I'm afraid there is a serious problem" followed by a pause allows the patient to prepare for the news. The patient will often ask for clarification when ready to listen to more. The doctor can then give further details and although euphemisms are occasionally helpful it is always best to use the word "cancer" at some stage to avoid confusion (see box 9.5). Some people believe that a patient's adjustment to diagnosis is made worse by using the word "cancer" but recent work has demonstrated that this is not the case.[13]

Once the bad news has been broken the doctor should check what the patient has absorbed and if necessary repeat any information that remains unclear. Diagrams, images or analogies can be used. Above all the doctor should try to take things at the patient's pace and accept that any patient will have a limited capacity to absorb details at such times. Acknowledging this and trying to make time available on another occasion is always desirable.

Box 9.5 Breaking bad news

- clarify the patient's understanding of the situation to judge the gap between their perception and reality
- elicit their coping strategy
- give them the news if they want to hear it
- explain slowly and give a warning shot before using the word cancer
- check understanding frequently

The use of simplified anatomical diagrams can be helpful to patients when explaining the result of investigations. Some patients appreciate being shown the radiological images during this process but, as with other aspects of breaking bad news, the doctor should first check the patient's coping strategy before displaying such images. A range exists between those who cope adequately by not allowing visual images of the cancer to come into their consciousness and those for whom active participation is very important. Images of the cancer make the disease more tangible; this can frighten some patients but for others it can act as a focus for their psychological battle. Conversely, some patients perceive their cancers as large and overwhelming and are greatly relieved to see that the cancer is much smaller in reality than they imagined, if this is the case.

Handling the responses

Crying. Many patients cry after hearing that they have cancer. The doctor should avoid looking embarrassed and should let the patient know that this is understandable and normal behaviour. Having tissues available and avoiding speaking whilst the patient recovers his or her composure shows empathy. Some doctors feel comfortable touching the patient but not all will feel this to be appropriate. It is a matter of personal style.

Anger. Anger is a fairly common response. The doctor can help discharge this by listening and letting patients give vent to their feelings. Remaining objective and calm is vital. It helps to remember that most patients are angry at the news rather than the doctor but it is common for the messenger to be blamed. Being defensive is rarely helpful.

Silence. Information may take a while to sink in. Silence can feel

---

Box 9.6 Responding to crying, silence and anger

- allow time for the bad news to sink in and responses to occur
- acknowledging the patient's position but avoid talking over these responses to save embarrassment
- defensiveness or irritation are unhelpful
- the patient is usually ready to re-engage with the doctor after a few minutes

---

awkward and it is tempting to rush in with further information. The doctor should wait for a signal that the patient is ready to re-engage in their conversation. The signal might be re-making eye contact or asking further questions. The doctor can empathise, eg, "It must be very hard to take this in" but a pitfall to avoid is jumping in with false hope (see box 9.6).

Identifying other concerns

After breaking the news and acknowledging the patient's feelings the doctor should establish the patient's concerns before any discussion of the future takes place. For example, a patient may express concern about uncontrolled symptoms such as pain. Re-assurance can be given that every effort will be made to give the best possible care and to help control troublesome symptoms. Some patients will ask about treatment. The role of surgery, radiotherapy or chemotherapy can then be addressed but it may be preferable to do this at a later interview if the patient seems unable to take in further details. A patient may have prior knowledge of some treatments but many myths abound and so careful explanation of likely side-effects is beneficial. Quoting inflated success rates for treatments should be avoided as it can lead to anger and bitterness later if they fail.

Box 9.7 Discussing prognosis

- identify any concerns that the patient has for the future
- be realistic when discussing any proposed treatments
- avoid giving specific time frames
- if the patient will ultimately die of their disease, offer to explain signs and symptoms of deterioration but avoid frightening details
- provide examples of what the patient can reasonably hope for as appropriate, eg, symptom control, short remissions or time at home

---

Discussing prognosis

Questions about survival are asked by many patients. When replying to the question "How long have I got?" it is best to avoid a specific prediction. Maguire and Faulkner have highlighted the problem of patients and their relatives pacing themselves according to the time that they believe they have left.[14] If the patient

---

Box 9.8 Common pitfalls

- inadequate time or information
- failure to elicit the patient's understanding of the situation and their coping strategy
- breaking the news at the doctor's rather than the patient's pace
- not allowing time for responses or questions
- platitudes and false re-assurances about the future
- allowing collusion with relatives
- allowing denial to remain unchallenged when it is causing difficulties for the patient and their relatives
- removing all hope

---

deteriorates sooner than anticipated they feel cheated and bitter at not achieving specific goals. An unexpected remission can be viewed as borrowed time and there may be no emotional and physical resources left to cope with this. It is better to acknowledge the uncertainty. Some patients are helped by a framework, for example, "Well, it may be months rather than years, but it is unlikely to be a few weeks". This should be followed by repeating the uncertainty of the situation. Occasionally patients or relatives interpret general guidance into specific numbers of weeks or months, no matter how vague the information they have been given.

It is vital at this point to state the aim of any treatment that is available and to emphasise the difference between a "treatment" and a "cure". If cure is not possible then this should be conveyed sensitively.

When confronted by the question "Am I going to die?" the doctor should remember that this is a brave question and try to be honest. A reply such as "It is likely that the cancer will shorten your life" is one option which allows the patient to ask for more details if they wish to explore this area further.

Some patients ask for guidance on how to recognise disease progression in themselves. The doctor should then describe the symptoms that they believe the patient may experience but avoid frightening details, eg, "You may notice that you are more short of breath or more easily tired". This is also another opportunity for the doctor to ask about any worries that the patient has about their future and to tackle each one separately. The memory of a relative who died in pain from cancer years ago may be a potent source of fear for the patient facing their own death (see box 9.7).

Closing the interview

The doctor should warn the patient that the interview is drawing to a close and ask the patient about any other possible worries or questions. Re-assurance about continuing support should be offered and plans made for another consultation soon. It should be remembered that coping strategies change and a patient who has been reluctant to hear bad news may be more ready to hear it at a later date. Details should be given of how the doctor can be contacted. Leaving a nurse to continue the discussion can help some patients but not all.

It is vital for teamwork that the doctor writes legibly what the patient has been told during the interview in the clinical notes. For example, "Patient told that he has stomach cancer and that it is very unlikely that he can be cured" is better and more specific than "diagnosis and prognosis discussed". Letters to general

---

Case history 9.1

A junior doctor on-call for the weekend is called to see a young woman who has had a definite carcinoma of the cervix diagnosed but has not yet been told of the diagnosis. The patient is asking what is wrong with her.

The doctor could:

- read the notes carefully to ensure that the correct information is understood
- explain to the patient who he is and that he will try to help
- sit with the patient, in private if possible, and find out what she understands about her symptoms and investigations
- ask the patient if she would like the doctor to explain the results but also ask if she wants a relative to be present
- break the news if she wants to know in the manner outlined in the text
- write in the notes exactly what has been discussed
- try to speak to the consultant's team when they are back on duty. It is unlikely that the doctor will be reproached if he has responded to the patient's wishes and broken the news in a sensitive way

---

practitioners and referring consultants should always include a clear statement about what the patient has been told. A brief phone call to the patient's general practitioner will be much appreciated as this allows the GP to check on the patient's emotional response and provide support for the patient and family in their own home. Most doctors find it stressful and upsetting to give bad news and, whenever possible it is helpful to allow a few minutes break before going onto the next task.

Difficult areas

Denial

Denial can be a useful coping mechanism when patients cannot adjust to the information given to them. It becomes a problem when it causes significant anguish for patients or relatives and if it stops patients themselves from dealing with important issues for family members.

A sensitive and assertive probing of patients' stories and confronting them with the incongruence between their symptoms and explanation may be enough to break the denial in an appropriate way. Patients can change from a position of denial to acceptance of cancer and opportunities for asking questions should be allowed at each consultation.

Case history 9.2

A middle aged man with lung cancer has been receiving chemotherapy but a recent CT scan demonstrates marked deterioration of his disease. He is waiting in out-patients to hear the result of the scan from the consultant.

The consultant could:

● introduce herself if she has not met the patient before
● check what the patient understands about his condition and how he perceives the effect of the treatment so far
● warn the patient that the scan is not as good as expected
● check that he wants more explanation
● explain the scan in detail if requested
● go on to discuss alternative management and future prognosis if the patient asks, or offer to see the patient at the next out-patient clinic to let the news sink in before discussing the future

---

Collusion with relatives

A conspiracy of silence can contribute to a lonely, isolated death if a patient is not given the opportunity of knowing the diagnosis. The strain on relatives of maintaining the "secret" can be immense. It is important to challenge collusion to spare the patient the anxiety and distress of isolation and to avoid a complicated bereavement for relatives, who were prevented from being open with the patient by their conspiracy.

An important ethical principle is that clinical information should be discussed with a patient first, and only then with the relatives if the patient has given permission for the doctor to do so. The reality is that doctors are sometimes requested by relatives not to tell patients bad news before the doctor has even had a chance to see the patient. Usually the relative expresses fears that the patient will not be able to cope with the news and will "give up" and they may be worried that the patient will be told bad news in a blunt manner.

In such situations, the doctor needs to be assertive whilst remaining approachable and re-assuring. Explaining the ethical position is often useful as it is not always known by the lay public. The doctor can also explain the difficulties that can be caused by a patient not knowing the diagnosis and can offer to carry out a discussion with the patient in as sensitive a way as possible. It is also helpful to point out to relatives that it is a natural response to become upset when hearing of a diagnosis of cancer but that many people do adjust to that knowledge. Finally, relatives should be re-assured that, if the patient indicates a clear desire not to be given bad news, this will be respected.

Cultural differences

Different cultural groups have different attitudes to disclosure of medical information. The doctor needs to be alert to this and be prepared to respect the patient's view. If there is also a language barrier and a close relative of the patient is asked to interpret, it is helpful to try and establish how comfortable the relative feels to do so. The doctor needs to be aware that the message conveyed to the patient may be altered by the interpreter because of differing traditions in what is considered acceptable practice. This is a complex area and requires more detailed analysis than is the scope of this chapter.

Case history 9.3

An elderly man with back pain has had a blood test performed by his general practitioner. Serum prostate-specific antigen was consistent with metastatic carcinoma of the prostate but the patient's wife has telephoned to say that he must not be told any bad news.

The general practitioner could:

- acknowledge the wife's concern for her husband and explain that the doctor will be sensitive
- outline the ethical position, ie, her husband has a right to know if he wants to but that the doctor will not force the information on him
- stress to the wife that it is best to be open about the situation now rather than risking the distrust of her husband if he found out at a later stage, eg, if symptoms became worse

When seeing that patient, the doctor could:

- check with the patient what he understands about the possible diagnosis
- ask whether he wants to know the implications of the blood tests and if he wants his wife present
- break the news if requested
- explain the potential treatments available if the patient indicates that they want the doctor to do so
- offer another appointment to see the patient with his wife if she was not present

1   Cassileth BR, Zupkis RV, Sutton-Smith K, March V. Information and participation preferences among cancer patients. *Ann Intern Med* 1980;**92**:832-6.

2   Blanchard CG, Labreque MS, Ruckdeschel JC, Blanchard ED. Information and decision making preferences of hospitalized adult cancer patients. *Soc Sci Med* 1988;**27**:1139-45.

3   Maguire P. Can communication skills be taught? *Br J Hosp Med* 1990;**43**:215-6.

4   Maguire P, Faulkner A. How to do it - improve counselling skills of doctors and nurses in cancer care. *BMJ* 1988;**297**:847-9.

5   McManus IC, Vincent CA, Thom S, Kidd J. How to do it - teaching communication skills to clinical students. *BMJ* 1993;**306**:1322-7.

6   Cassidy S, Burns G, Smearden K.. *The cancer journey* (video cassette). Professional Video Productions c/o British Gas plc, South Eastern, Katherine St, Croydon CG9 1JU.

7   Faulkner A, Maguire P. In: *Talking to cancer patients and their families.* Oxford: Oxford University Press, 1995; pp 187-94.

8   Calman K. Quality of life in cancer patients - an hypothesis. *J Med Ethics* 1984;**10**:125-7.

9   Buckman R. *How to break news.* London: Pan Books, 1994; pp 11-2.

10 Maguire P, Faulkner A. How to do it - communicate with cancer patients. 1. Handling bad news and difficult questions. *BMJ* 1988;**297**:907-9.

11 Tattersall MH, Butow PN, Griffin AM, Dunn SM. The take home message: patients prefer consultation audiotapes to summary letters. *J Clin Oncal* 1994;**12**:1305-11.

12 Hogbin B, Fallowfield L. Getting it taped: the bad news consultation with cancer patients. *Br J Hosp Med* 1989;**41**:330-3.

13 Dunn SM, Patterson PJ, Butow PN, Smart HH, McCarthy WH, Tattersall MH. Cancer by another name - a randomised trial of the effectiveness of euphemism and uncertainty in communicating with cancer patients. *J Clin Oncol* 1993;**11**:989-96.

14 Maguire P, Faulkner A. How to do it - communicate with cancer patients. 2. Handling uncertainty, collusion and denial. *BMJ* 1988;**297**:972-4.

10 Dealing with the "difficult" patient

SAM SMITH

It is said that the first step doctors must take in managing difficult patients is to accept their own negative feelings towards them.[1,2] Otherwise, in the effort to escape them, needless referrals and unnecessary investigations may be made or ordered. Patients described as difficult by their doctors have been shown to attend more frequently with acute and chronic problems, to be prescribed more medication, have more investigations ordered for them, and to be referred more often for a second opinion.[3,4] The fat folders of such patients[5] testify to the amount of medical work generated, and many attempts have been made to define the characteristics of so-called problem patients.[4,6-8] It is increasingly recognised, however, that this extra and often clinically unnecessary work is a product of the doctor–patient relationship, for which both parties have a responsibility.[2,9-12] Indeed, the outcome of consultations with patients in general, depends on demonstrable aspects of the behaviour of both doctors and patients. This is true both in terms of clinical parameters,[13] and in terms of patient compliance and satisfaction.[14-16]

Rather than the characteristics of problem patients alone, therefore, what demands attention is how characteristics of both patient and doctor shape, and are shaped by, the doctor–patient interaction. Thus, an approach which explores the difficulties of the clinical transaction itself, rather than the supposed failings of the problem patient, is likely to prove more fruitful.[17] Social forces which influence the attitudes and expectations of both doctors and patients, must also be given consideration. These influences are not

101

necessarily harmonious, for whilst there is often a productive reciprocity of doctor and patient roles, this cannot be assumed.[18] As well as conforming to the pressures of social norms, doctors and patients develop as unique individuals, and bring personal and idiosyncratic attributes to the clinical transaction. Aspects of personality can dramatically effect the process and outcome of the clinical transaction[17,19]

These themes will be explored in this chapter with the aim of reframing the problem of the difficult patient, and thereby going some way towards dispelling it. Any improvement in the quality and outcome of clinical transactions with such patients might be judged by the evaporation of negative feelings, and fewer unnecessarily fat folders.

Characteristics of problem patients

Historically, strict medical criteria for identifying problem patients have not been uniformly employed.[3] They are more often women, and complain of ill-defined somatic symptoms which fluctuate over time and seem to have no organic basis.[2] Whilst consuming disproportionate amounts of healthcare they appear to gain little benefit from it. They are capable of kindling aversion, fear, despair or even downright malice in their doctors.[6] Such powerful feelings fuel the process by which doctors attach to these patients such unflattering epithets as heartsink,[7] black holes,[8] crocks or turkeys,[12] and many more besides. Stereotyping, however, may prejudice the range of responses brought to bear on a problem, especially if the stereotype is a stigmatising label.

Box 10.1 Demographic characteristics of difficult patients

- older
- more often divorced or widowed
- more often female
- attend more frequently
- more acute problems
- more chronic problems
- more medications
- more x rays, blood tests and referrals
- have fat folders
- no less provider continuity

Problem patients are often said to display abnormal illness behaviour, somatise, or to suffer from a personality disorder.

Abnormal illness behaviour

According to the biomedical model, symptoms are the subjectively experienced consequences of physical or psychiatric disease. Furthermore, in Western medical epistemology, it is held that there is a correspondence and association between changes in the body, and states of mind and behaviour.[20] Symptoms, therefore, ought only to exist in the presence of disease, and should provoke the patient to seek appropriate medical help. It has become obvious, however, that people experience and respond to their symptoms in many different ways. To account for this fact, Mechanic developed the concept of illness behaviour.[21] The concept was extended by Pilowski to encompass the presentation of symptoms in the absence of disease, or out of proportion to the degree of physical pathology.

Patients who present with trivial or unfounded somatic complaints can, by this account, still find their place within medical rationality if deemed to be displaying abnormal illness behaviour.[22] A short step further, and such modes of presentation can be assigned a psychiatric origin, and thus be firmly reclaimed by the medical model. This doctor/disease centred endeavour has been increasingly criticised.[18]

Somatisation

Somatising patients are defined as those who frequently complain of physical symptoms that either lack demonstrable organic bases or are judged to be grossly in excess of what one would expect on the grounds of objective medical findings.[23] Such patients are often labelled difficult by their doctors. As a concept, like abnormal illness behaviour, somatisation bridges the mind/body and disease/illness dualism that is so challenged by much of patient behaviour. The determinants of somatisation are not entirely clear and may depend on cultural or familial factors.[23] When compared to patients who present problems in more psychosocial terms (psychologisers), somatisers tend to be less depressed, report lower levels of social dissatisfaction, less social stress and less depressed, report lower levels of social dissatisfaction, less social stress and less dependence on relatives.

They are more likely to have an unsympathetic attitude towards mental illness and less likely to consult a doctor about psychological symptoms. They are more likely to have received medical in-patient care as an adult before they had consulted their doctor with their current illness.[24] In spite of these findings, there is a clear link between somatisation and psychiatric illness, especially depression,[24] and patients who present somatically are more likely to be misdiagnosed as having a physical illness by their doctors.[25] Somatisation is often used interchangeably with concepts such as hypochondriasis and hysteria. These terms, however, are often employed pejoratively, rather than as reliable diagnostic terms. It is doubtful whether somatisation itself achieves the status of a diagnosis, for it is often observed, even if only transiently, as part of the normal presentation of illness.[22]

Box 10.2 Personality disorder

- often associated with various degrees of subjective distress and with problems in social functioning and performance

- care should be taken in applying this term diagnostically

- not all problem patients have a diagnosable personality disorder

- some doctors may have a diagnosable personality disorder

Personality disorder

Those who suffer from disordered personalities, be they patients or doctors, are often difficult to deal with. The definition of personality disorder[26] is based in part on this very fact. It is a complex subject and only one or two points will be made here. A feature of personality disorder involves the prominent and habitual deployment of rigid mechanisms of psychological defence. Such defences develop to protect the mind against the psychological effects of sustained adverse circumstances during the early development of the personality.[17] Their effect is to distort a person's perception of themselves and others in ways which interfere significantly with straightforward communication and the capacity to seek and receive help (see below). By no means all problem patients, however, satisfy strict criteria for a diagnosable personality disorder.

Characteristics of doctors

By virtue of their medical training, together with aspects of their personalities, doctors develop a particular style of relating to patients and their problems. For an individual doctor, this style seems to be remarkably constant from consultation to consultation[36] and has been typified in numerous ways,[14-16, 27-29, 36] One important dimension that distinguishes doctors is how doctor-centred òr patient-centred they are. This depends on how far doctors adhere to a strict medical model as opposed to a more psychosocial or counselling approach involving an attempt to see the problem in the patient's own terms. Another observable dimension is the capacity to tolerate uncertainty and the willingness to take risks.[29] In terms of the patients they treat, doctors characteristically rate as most difficult to help those who: attend frequently; show more emotional distress; have symptoms unexplained by organic disease; have chronic organic disease together with severe psychological problems; and those with chronic disease for which medical treatment is ineffective.[30]

It should be remembered that the personal characteristics of an

---

Case history 10.1

Following her husband's death from a heart attack, Mrs A herself developed chest pains. A diagnosis of angina was made. She became neurotically anxious about her heart and was admitted to hospital several times with chest pain. Myocardial infarction was never confirmed. She frequently consulted her general practitioner, who came to dread her visits, and her treatment was change many times. Following her last admission, an exercise electrocardiogram was arranged which was completely normal. When told this she was at first disbelieving, then became depressed. As part of the treatment of depression she was able to address her fears and the unresolved grief after losing her husband. Her chest pains did not return.

Comment
Mrs A became a difficult patient for her general practitioner because of her anxiety, her failure to respond to treatment, and his own doubt about the potentially life-threatening diagnosis. The equivocal outcome of her hospital admissions compounded a process of somatic fixation. This perpetuated Mrs A's psychological defence of denial and avoidance in the face of her husband's death.

---

individual doctor can contribute as much to the difficulty of a clinical transaction as those of the patient.

Doctor–patient interaction

Those aspects of patients and doctors discussed so far obviously fall short of a complete and relevant characterisation. They are important, however, because they contribute to the styles in which patients present and doctors respond to illness (box 10.3). If styles are not compatible, this may complicate the clinical transaction. A medically oriented doctor, for example, might have difficulty dealing with an emotional presentation of psychosocial problems.

Box 10.3 Doctors' styles

- doctors' styles can affect the outcome of clinical transactions

- task-oriented styles, where information is exchanged, lead to better compliance

- styles including social and emotional exchange lead to greater satisfaction

- doctors' styles tend to be fixed

- problems can arise when the consulting styles of patient and doctor conflict

---

A patient whose idiom of self expression is primarily somatic, may have difficulty cooperating with a psychosocial enquiry.[17] Hall has shown that the outcome of the doctor–patient interaction, in terms of patient compliance, is favoured by an informative and task orientated style. Satisfaction is more related to the amount of socioemotional exchange.[15] Better health outcomes in terms of physiological measurements and functional capacity result from interactions in which there is: more control by patients; more expression of emotion (positive or negative) by either doctor or patient; and more information sought by patients and given by doctors.[13] On the other hand, doctor centred interactions, as Grol has found, are associated with more prescription of symptomatic medication and poorer psychosocial care.[27] The presentation of somatic symptoms within the context of a rigidly applied medical model can lead to somatic fixation and over-medicalisation.[31]

Public and personal domains

The public domain

Health benefits and expectations, for both patient and doctor, are largely constructed through either formal—as in this case of medical training—or informal social practices. Such practices result in the conventional roles enacted by doctor and patient within the clinical transaction. Each role implies certain attitudes and entails certain responsibilities, such as establishing a diagnosis, prescribing medication, and cooperating and complying with

---

Box 10.4 Public and personal domains

- the doctor–patient interaction is pursued on two levels
- the public domain encompasses the attitudes, expectations, and responsibilities defined by social roles, including clinical work
- the personal domain encompasses the level of interaction determined by aspects of the individual personalities of doctor and patient
- style is a combination of public and personal influences
- the domains interact
- failures in clinical transactions can become apparent in one domain, but originate in the other

---

treatment. The clinical tasks of the transaction, including negotiating and agreeing appropriate goals, constitute the public domain of doctor–patient interaction.[17] As Armstrong has pointed out, there is not always a cosy reciprocity between the roles of doctor and patient, and patients may not present with illnesses which comfortably conform to the medical model. This does not mean, however, that they cannot account for their symptoms in rational terms, even if they are not the terms of medical rationality.[18] Some effort must be made, therefore, to ensure a shared understanding of problems and explanations. In this respect it should be acknowledged that the performance of the patient role demands a level of psychosocial accomplishment and maturity that some patients do not achieve. Furthermore, any such capacity is likely to be undermined by the effects of illness itself.

The personal domain

As well as being pursued on the level of the public domain, clinical transactions necessarily involve the interaction of doctor and patient as individual personalities. At this level reactions to the other person are immediate and can fluctuate rapidly. Such reactions may generate emotions reaching awareness, but they may motivate behaviour unconsciously. For example, doctors are, at least to some extent, a self selecting group pursuing a vocation. Their motivation is likely to lead them to act in the service of patients and thus sustains the straightforward performance of the clinical transaction. At at personal level, however, care provided may be offered as if it were a gift to the patient. Should this gift of care be rejected or discounted by the patient doctors may be open to hurt or disappointment, and may feel less well disposed towards their patients as a consequence. Patients are often willing to be and genuinely are grateful, but some may have personal difficulty in receiving gifts. Others may regard any care provided more as a right than a gift.

Case history 10.2

Dr Z was a committed general practitioner who worked hard on behalf of her patients. Mr B, a young man, attended frequently with vague somatic symptoms and fatigue. Routine tests were normal and Dr Z concentrated on counselling and medication for depression. Mr B improved initially and seemed grateful, but before long his symptoms returned, and nothing seemed to help. On one occasion he brought back his unfinished medication describing it as useless. Dr Z was surprised at her sudden dislike for this patient, but concealing her irritation she said she would refer Mr B to a psychiatrist.

Comment

Mr B's rejection of Dr Z's treatment aroused hostility, which although concealed, may have prompted the decision to refer. This, in turn, may have been experienced by Mr B as a rejection. Acknowledging her feelings to herself, Dr Z might more productively have discussed the apparent stalemate they had reached observing, in a spirit of enquiry, the fact that nothing seemed to help.

Transference and countertransference

The circumstances and relationships of early development are inevitably beset by hardship and frustration to some degree. As a result people acquire patterns of psychological defences, and accumulate unresolved emotional conflicts, of which they are mostly unaware. These defences and conflicts remain to be erected or re-enacted in the context of current relationships via processes of transference and countertransference.[17] In some circumstances, such as when faced by a patient experienced as particularly difficult, it is as if these emotional residues are re-activated. A well disposed attitude may then be displaced by strong negative feelings, sometimes amounting to hate.[6,32-34] Such unwelcome emotions may be repressed, but at the risk of finding unconscious expression in punitive, neglectful, or rejecting responses towards patients. Strong positive, especially sexual, feelings can equally distort professional attitudes and behaviour, in different, but no less inappropriate ways.

People who have suffered severe and sustained adversity in early life, perhaps physical or sexual abuse in childhood, are likely to develop extreme and rigid defences as a consequence. Whilst internalising their experience as victims, they may, in an attempt to defend themselves against feelings of powerlessness and helplessness, also have internalised aspects of the powerful abuser.

Case history 10.3

Mr C seemed an aggressive and resentful young man. He had been known to shout at the receptionists and nurses in the hospital clinic he had attended for some time with a chronic illness. During one visit Sister Y, the nurse in charge, took him to task and in the heat of argument told him that he was just like her teenage son. Mr C responded by saying she was just like his mother.

Comment

It is, of course, appropriate and legitimate to place limits on acceptable behaviour. In this instance emotional conflicts arising in family systems breached the boundary of the professional nurse/patient system. Mr C's attitude in the clinic was fuelled by the ingrained resentment of his treatment by his parents. Sister Y's reaction was aggravated by ongoing problems with her own son. The interactive effect exacerbated matters leading to Sister Y's confrontation of Mr C. Limits imposed one-sidedly in the heat of an argument are unlikely to succeed. A quieter, more reflective approach might have been more effective, with an attempt to understand the underlying emotional problems. Particular attention should be paid to boundary issues.

The theme of victim/victimiser can thus come to dominate their relationships with others, including their doctors. When such a patient, with a strong sense of self as a victim, presents to a doctor, the doctor may be drawn unwittingly into enacting the victimiser. The result is a self-fulfilling prophecy in which the dominant experience of the patient's life is repeated.[17] The feelings generated in such circumstances represent a powerful form of covert communication which if understood, can illuminate the emotional predicament of the patient.[6] When things go wrong in a clinical transaction, therefore, it is not always a result of misdiagnosis or inadequate medication, or the awkwardness or stupidity of the difficult patient. It may also be a reflection of the acting out of personal and interpersonal conflicts by doctor, patient, or both.

Straightforward and complicated clinical transactions

A clinical transaction is straightforward when the interaction between doctor and patient, at both public and personal levels, proceeds at least relatively harmoniously to achieve an acceptable and appropriate outcome. When the process or outcome of a transaction is either unacceptable or inappropriate, in more than a trivial or transient way, the transaction has become complicated.[17] It can be tempting to locate the complication, often with apparent justification, within the psychopathology of the "problem patient". But whatever the personality of the patient (or the doctor for that matter) the complication itself emerges only in the context of the clinical transaction, and derives from the interaction between patient and doctor. Its origins are therefore more productively sought within this interaction, paying particular attention to how public and personal domains influence one another.

Systems

The theory of systems is widely applicable, and adopting a systemic perspective can help to re-frame the problem of difficult patients. Problems which derive from applying the medical model too narrowly can be avoided by adopting a biopsychosocial model.[35] According to such a model the human organism constitutes but one level in a natural hierarchy of systems ranging from the atomic to the cultural. These systems are linked by flows of information in the hierarchy which are different in nature at different levels; molecular at the level of the synapse, symbolic at the level of human language. Regulatory, homeostatic, and adaptive processes operate within and between systems. A particular disease may exert its primary effect at one level, but through the transmission and feedback of information, also affect other levels in the hierarchy. Such a perspective inclines towards interpretation of illness and disease in multifactorial, holistic and patient centered terms, rather than unitary causes and effects.

The clinical transaction involving an individual doctor and patient, can also be viewed as a system within the hierarchy of systems of healthcare. As individuals doctor and patient belong simultaneously to overlapping systems such as families. Events in one system influence, and are influenced by, events in other systems. For example, the decision to limit costs taken at one level of the healthcare hierarchy can effect the interaction of patient and doctor at the level of the clinical transaction. It is well to remember, when in the grip of a difficult encounter with a patient, that contributions to that difficulty may emanate from conflicts belonging more properly to another related system.[17]

Dealing with the difficult patient

Preventive measures: monitoring the clinical transaction

Becoming aware of and accepting negative feelings towards a patient can enable the doctor to avoid reacting in counter-productive ways. As discussed, negative feelings may be roused in doctors when: patients present illnesses that do not fit the medical model; medical and lay explanations of disease conflict; patients fail to comply with treatments or fail to respond to them; or when in some other respect patients fail to play the expected patient role. Patients may be unhappy with their doctors if they: do not listen; do not provide information; are incompetent; or do not engage emotionally with them in an appropriate way. Factors such as these are open to scrutiny because they lie predominantly within the public domain of the clinical transaction, and efforts can be made to remedy them.

More subtle influences on the doctor–patient interaction can be difficult to guard against. People unconsciously perceive and react to others on the basis of past important relationships and events, to a greater or lesser degree, and may project a role for them that may be grossly distorted and inaccurate. Negative feelings may be the result of being cast in a role that feels uncomfortable. Such a role may be incompatible with the view that doctors or patients have of themselves, or with an appropriate, professional doctor–patient relationship. For instance, patients sometimes over-idealise their doctors such that they can do no wrong. Alternatively, they may manifestly mistrust anything the doctor has to offer. Via similar psychological mechanisms doctors may fail to respect their patients sufficiently, perhaps adopting an infantilising approach, or treating any misunderstanding as evidence for the stupidity of the patient. Factors such as these lie within the personal domain of doctor–patient interaction and are consequently often more obvious to others than to the participants themselves. Discussion with colleagues can be extremely helpful, especially if based on consultations which have been videotaped. Skill in monitoring the transaction on the personal level involves becoming aware of any out-of-place feelings, attitudes or behaviour that arise. These may represent the earliest clues that all may not be well. Norton and Smith emphasise the importance of recognising how public and personal domains interact. Even though an unsatisfactory outcome of a clinical transaction may obviously lie in the public domain, such as a failure to comply with treatment, the cause, such as a failure of trust, may lie in the personal domain. They describe the use of a transaction window as an aid in deciding where, how, and why clinical transactions have become complicated.[17]

Case history 10.4

At a practice meeting held to discuss problem cases, a partner commented on Dr X's management of a depressed patient, Mr D, after watching a videotaped consultation. Both appeared dejected. The partner pointed out to Dr X that no mention had been made of Mr D's recent referral to hospital for investigation of a potentially malignant condition. A letter in the notes indicated that, in fact, Mr D had failed to attend when sent for. At their next meeting Dr X took the matter up with Mr D and discovered that Mr D had not told his wife and family about this condition because he felt everything was so pointless.

Comment

Dr X had experienced Mr D's depression as burdensome. Possibly the contagious feelings of futility had contributed to Dr X's neglect of the important matter of the referral. The practice meeting served to break the stalemate. Involving the family resulted in Mr D attending hospital, and an overall improvement in his mental state.

Reparative measures

Some patients, despite the most sincere and committed efforts of their doctors, seem to be beyond the reach of medical help, and yet persist in seeking it. In a few cases, some authors conclude that time is more profitably spent with other patients.[7,8] In many cases more positive action can be taken (see box 10.5).[2,7,8,17] It may be worthwhile to conduct a thorough psychosocial enquiry, involving other professionals where appropriate. Sharing problems with colleagues can both lighten the burden and be a source of valuable insight into the stalemate that so often exists. Other members of the primary healthcare team and the practice staff should be involved in order to develop a consistent approach towards such patients. These measures complement the monitoring of clinical transactions described above.

Box 10.5 Reparative measures

- review the notes
- review and re-assess doctors' and patients' feelings and behaviour, for evidence of unwanted transference and counter-transference effects (consider using videotapes)
- review the possibility of conflicting influences from related systems
- agree, list and prioritise problems
- set realistic limits on expectations of the delivery and outcome of care
- consider treatment contracts
- involve other family members
- discuss with partners and other members of practice staff

---

1   Cohen J. Diagnosis and management of problem patients in general practice. *J R Coll Gen Pract* 1987;**37**:51.

2   Corney RH, Strathdee G, King M, Williams P, Sharp D, Pelosi AJ. Managing the difficult patient: practical suggestions from a study day. *J R Coll Gen Pract* 1988;**38**:349-52.

3   McGaghie WC, Whitenack RH. A scale of measurement of the problem patient labelling process. *J Nerv Ment Dis* 1982;**170**:598-604.

4   John C, Schwenk TL, Roi LD, Cohen M. Medical care and the demographic characteristics of "difficult" patients. *J Fam Pract* 1987;**24**:607-10.

5   Schrire S. Frequent attenders - a review. *Fam Pract* 1986;**3**:272-5.

6   Groves JE. Taking care of the hateful patient. *N Engl J Med* 1978;**298**:883-5.

7   O'Dowd TC. Five years of heartsink patients in general practice. *BMJ* 1988;**297**:528-30.

8   Gerrard TJ, Riddell JD. Difficult patients: black holes and secrets. *BMJ* 1988;**297**:530-2.

9   Anstett R. The difficult patient and the physician–patient relationship. *J Fam Pract* 1980;11:281-6.
10 Baughan DM, Revicki D, Nieman LZ. Management of problem patients with multiple chronic diseases. *J Fam Pract* 1983;17:233-9.
11 Crutcher JE, Bass MJ. The difficult patient and the troubled physician. *J Fam Pract* 1980;11:933-8.
12 Kuch JH, Schuman SS, Curry HB. The problem patient and the problem doctor or do quacks make crocks? *J Fam Pract* 1977; 5: 647-53.
13 Horder J, Moore GT. The consultation and health outcomes. *Br J Gen Pract* 1990;40:442-3.
14 Hall JA, Roter DL, Katz NR. Task versus socioemotional behaviour in physicians. *Med Care* 1987;25:399-412.
15 Hall JA, Roter DL, Katz NR. Meta-analysis of correlates of provider behaviour in medical encounters. *Med Care* 1988;26:657-75.
16 Savage R, Armstrong D. Effect of a general practitioner's style on patient's satisfaction. *BMJ* 1990;301:968-70.
17 Norton K, Smith S. *Problems with patients: managing complicated transactions.* Cambridge: Cambridge University Press, 1994.
18 Armstrong D. Illness behaviour revisited. In: Lacey JH, Sturgeon DA, eds. *Proceedings of the 15th European Conference on Psychosomatic Research.* London: John Libby & Co Ltd, 1986; pp 115-9.
19 Balint M. *The doctor, his patient, and the illness.* New York: International Universities Press, 1957.
20 Fabrega H. The concept of somatization as a cultural and historical product of Western medicine. *Psychosom Med* 1990;52:653-72.
21 Mechanic D. The concept of illness behaviour. *J Chronic Dis* 1962;15:189-94.
22 Pilowski I. Abnormal illness behaviour. *Br J Med Psychol* 1969; 42: 347-51.
23 Lipowski ZJ. Somatization: the concept and its clinical application. *Am J Psychiatry* 1989;145:1358-68.
24 Bridges K, Goldberg D, Evans B, Sharpe T. Determinants of somatization in primary care. *Psychol Med* 1991;21:473-83.
25 Katon W, Kleinman A, Rosen G. Depression and somatisation, a review. *Am J Med* 1982;72:127-35.
26 World Health Organization. *ICD-10 Classification of mental and behavioural disorders. Clinical descriptions and diagnostic guidelines.* Geneva, WHO, 1992.
27 Grol R, de Maeseneer J, Whitfield M, Mokkink H. Disease-centred versus patient-centred attitudes: comparison of general practitioners in Britain, Belgium and The Netherlands. *Fam Pract* 1990;7:100-3.
28 Bucks RS, Williams A, Whitfield MJ, Routh DA. Towards a typology of general practitioners' attitudes in general practice. *Soc Sci Med* 1990;30:537-47.
29 Calnan M. Images of general practice: the perceptions of the doctor. *Soc Sci Med* 1988;27:579-86.
30 Sharpe M, Mayou R, Seagroatt V, *et al.* Why do doctors find some patients difficult to help? *Q J Med* 1994;87:187-93.
31 Grol R. *To heal or to harm: the prevention of somatic fixation in general practice.* R Coll Gen Pract Monogr, 1981.
32 Winnicott DW. Hate in the countertransference. In: *Through paediatrics to psycho-analysis.* London: Hogarth Press & The Institute of Psycho-Analysis, 1987.
33 Prodgers A. On hating the patient. *Br J Psychother* 1991;8:144-54.
34 Adler G. Helplessness in the helpers. *Br J Med Psychol* 1972;45:315-26.
35 Engel GL. A unified concept of health and disease. *Perspect Biol Med* 1960;3:459-85.
36 Byrnee PS, Long BEL. *Doctors talking to patients.* R Coll Gen Pract Monogr, 1984.

11 Discussing cardiopulmonary resuscitation with the patient and relatives

KEVIN STEWART

In the United Kingdom there is confusion about how much patients and relatives should be involved in decisions about cardiopulmonary resuscitation (CPR).[1-10]

This chapter aims to give precise guidelines for doctors working in general hospitals in the UK, based on ethical and legal principles, which will help them identify:

- when they are obliged to obtain patients' consent before making Do Not Resuscitate (DNR) decisions

- when they can make DNR decisions without consent

- when to involve patients' relatives in discussions

- what information they should give to patients

- what to do if there are disagreements with patients or relatives

- how this might change in the future

Background

In the United States policies have existed for many years which require doctors to obtain patients' consent before making DNR decisions.[11] If patients are unable to participate in decisions then there is legal provision for relatives to act on their behalf. These policies emphasise respect for patient autonomy in medical decision making, although there is evidence that American doctors do not always practice in accordance with them.[11]

In the UK many hospitals did not have written resuscitation policies until recently;[3] the traditional view was that these were unnecessary, since British patients were more likely to trust their doctors to decide on their behalf.[12] Consultants usually made decisions without informing patients, to save them from undue distress. This has subsequently been called "indefensibly paternalistic"[11] but probably represents widespread practice.

Recent interest in CPR was stimulated by the 1991 report of the Health Service Commissioner,[13] who upheld a complaint from a patient's son about a DNR decision made on his mother by a junior doctor. He expressed surprise that a written CPR policy seemed to be "something of a novelty" and suggested that hospitals should develop policies. Guidelines from the British Medical Association and the Royal College of Physicians of London[1,2] will help hospitals establish policies, but they do not give specific advice about discussing resuscitation with patients and relatives, or what to do if there is disagreement. Doyal and Wilsher's guidelines[14] are likely to be of more practical benefit, and they recognise that (unlike the United States) relatives do not have a legal right to make decisions on behalf of incompetent patients. Recently, in the first legal challenge to a DNR order in the UK, the High Court upheld the right of a hospital to make DNR decisions and commended the hospital involved for basing its policy on the BMA guidelines.[15]

There have been no large British studies addressing this subject although there have been a number of smaller ones, mostly in elderly patients.[5-10,16] Many of these have limitations and highlight the confusion that exists among patients, their relatives, their doctors and the investigators themselves. The authors of one paper claimed, quite incorrectly, that the defence organisations advised doctors that they were always obliged to perform CPR if patients requested it.[8] The defence organisations later refuted this.[17]

Most British studies have interviewed those who were about to be discharged from hospital or who were out-patients.[5-8,10] CPR decisions need to be made at the time of admission; patients who survive to discharge and are able to discuss resuscitation at that time are not a representative group. The patients in whom decisions are most needed, of course, are those who die in hospital. Other groups where decisions may be difficult are those with dementia and those who are very ill at the time of admission, but these patients are excluded from most studies. Gunasekera[6] was

116

only able to interview 136 out of 716 (19%) patients initially considered suitable for his study, and Potter et al[9] attempted to interview all elderly patients on admission but excluded just over half because they were too ill or too confused. Likewise, Bruce-Jones and colleagues had to exclude about two thirds of those initially thought suitable for their study.[16] Even patients awaiting discharge are not always well enough to participate in discussions; about a quarter are excluded, mostly because of confusion.[5,10]

Most studies have given inadequate information about CPR and then tried to determine patients' preferences. Many patients think that CPR is usually successful and, on this basis, want it for themselves.[5,6,9,10] Patients' main source of information about CPR appears to be television drama[5] but this unfortunately seems to portray resuscitation attempts as usually being successful. Diem and colleagues[18] found that about two thirds of patients having CPR attempts on the American television programmes which they surveyed seemed to survive to leave hospital. CPR is, however, usually unsuccessful, with survival to leave hospital usually being in the range 10 to 20%. Murphy and colleagues[19] have demonstrated the importance of giving patients a detailed explanation of CPR, including realistic information about the expected outcome. 41% of their elderly American patients initially wanted CPR but this fell to 22% when the true outcome was explained. 56% of Liddle and colleagues[10] patients thought that CPR was usually successful, as did 58% of Mead and Turnbull's.[5] In both studies only a general explanation of CPR was given without reference to outcome. Potter and colleagues[9] specifically avoided discussing outcome, and in three other studies it is unclear what patients were told.[6-8] If, in clinical practice, these investigators had tried to obtain informed consent for DNR decisions on the basis of the information given in their studies, it would almost certainly have been invalid.

Many patients would not want to be resuscitated if they had severe physical or mental impairment, especially dementia. 75% of Robertson's patients[20] would not want CPR if they were so confused that they could not recognise family and friends, and this is confirmed in other studies.[6-10]

There is evidence that some British patients may prefer doctors to act in a paternalistic way. Between 14% and 65% of patients[5,6,10,16] think that the final decision about CPR should be the doctor's and between 23% and 34%[5,8] do not want their relatives involved in decisions. Some authors[5,9] advocate discussing CPR routinely with all elderly patients on admission to hospital, even though the evidence is that this is impractical and may not be what patients want. Potter and colleagues[9] had to exclude those patients who were most likely to require resuscitation decisions (the very ill and those with dementia) from discussing them. Mead and Turnbull[5] support a policy of routine discussions with all competent patients, but their study does not show that this is what patients want; 35% of their patients wanted to be involved in discussions, 14% did not, and 51% had no preference. Only 28% of Liddle's patients[10] said they wanted to discuss resuscitation at the time of hospital admission. Heller and colleagues instituted such a policy but[21] found that their intentions were misunderstood by the patient, relatives and local MP, and subsequently misrepresented by the media. In practice doctors discuss CPR with relatives occasionally[7] but rarely with patients[11] even if they profess to be strong believers in the principle.

Overall, these studies suggest that some patients want to be more involved in decisions but there may still be many who do not, or who want to leave this to their doctors, and others who do not want their relatives involved. There are practical difficulties, since those who most require resuscitation decisions are those who are also unlikely to be able to participate in discussions.

Ethical and moral principles

There are four ethical principles which govern resuscitation decisions.[14,22]

These are:

● respect for patient autonomy

● beneficence

● non-maleficence

● justice

Autonomy is the ability to think, decide and then act on such thought, freely and without hindrance.[22] Respect for autonomy implies that doctors treat patients in accordance with their informed choices, even if this conflicts with the doctor's beliefs.

Beneficence refers to the need to do good, and *non-maleficence* to the need to avoid harm. These imply that treatment must be thought to be likely to succeed or that the potential benefits must outweigh the potential risks.

The principle of *justice* refers to the doctor's duty to society as a whole. Using scarce resources to continue aggressive treatment for a terminally ill patient is potentially depriving others of the treatment.

Competence and incompetence

In order to be legally and ethically competent to consent to treatment, patients must possess the following requirements, and demonstrate them repeatedly and consistently over time:[23-25]

- understand a simple explanation of their condition, its likely outcome and any proposed treatment

- be able to reason consistently about specific goals of treatment

- choose to act on the basis of such reasoning

- communicate their choice and the reason for it

- understand the consequences of their choice.

Competence to discuss one issue does not necessarily imply competence to discuss others.[23,24] Competence can be impaired as a result of a psychiatric condition (dementia, toxic confusional state) or because of a physical condition. Patients in a coma are clearly incompetent but so too may be those who are in severe pain, dyspnoeic, or dehydrated.

Consent and confidentiality

Consent to treatment

Competent adults have the right to give or refuse consent to be examined or treated[26] and must also give consent if doctors are considering withholding or withdrawing life sustaining or life saving treatment, which would otherwise be considered part of normal medical treatment.[14,23]

Consent should be informed;[26] the patient must be told the likely outcome of treatment and potential risks. Consent for DNR decisions does not have to be explicit[14] but can be implied by statements given repeatedly and consistently by competent patients refusing life prolonging treatment in general. Relatives are commonly asked to sign consent forms for incompetent patients but, although this is good clinical practice, it has no basis in English law at present.[23] Doctors have an obligation to make clinical decisions on behalf of incompetent patients, in the patients' best interests.[23]

Confidentiality

Doctors have an ethical and legal obligation of confidentiality to patients.[26] There are circumstances when this can legitimately be broken, but doctors usually require permission from patients to disclose information about them to third parties. Incompetent patients have the same rights to confidentiality as competent ones. It is common practice in the UK for doctors to discuss patients' clinical conditions with relatives[7,24,27] and permission to do this is often implied rather than sought explicitly. If a patient is competent then it is good practice to seek permission before discussing clinical details with relatives.

Reasons for making DNR decisions

DNR decisions are made for several reasons:[1,2,14,28]

1 Refusal—a competent, fully informed patient asks to be excluded from CPR.

2 Poor quality of life after CPR—CPR has a measurable chance of success but the quality of life after resuscitation is likely to be so poor that it is unacceptable to the patient. It is the patient's perception of his or her quality of life which is important, not that of the doctors or family.

3 Futility—the chances of the patient surviving CPR are so low that it can be regarded as futile. This is a clinical decision which does not need to involve the patient, and there is no obligation to attempt CPR in these circumstances.

Patients with disseminated malignancy, prolonged hypotension, septicaemia or severe cardiac failure virtually never survive CPR[11,29] and those with pneumonia, advanced renal impairment or who had such severe chronic illness before admission that they were homebound have a very low survival rate.

There is considerable debate in the United States about the definition and scope of futility, and some authors argue that doctors can never be completely certain that CPR is futile.[11,31] Doctors in the UK would probably take a more pragmatic approach.[11] They may be attracted to the proposals of Blackhall[29] who notes that the chances of surviving CPR in a persistent vegetative state (which many people would regard as less desirable than death) are 1-2%, and CPR should be regarded as futile if the chances of surviving are less than this.

Circumstances when it is necessary to discuss DNR decisions with patients

- if a competent patient indicates that he wishes to discuss CPR.[14]

- if a DNR decision is being considered for a competent patient on the grounds of poor quality of life (and CPR is thought likely to have some chance of success). Informed consent must usually be obtained although this can be implied rather than explicit,[23] and there are occasions when this general rule can be broken (see below).

Circumstances when it is not necessary to discuss DNR decisions with patients

- when a patient is judged to be incompetent by the doctor who is making the DNR decision[25]

- if a DNR decision is being considered for a competent patient on the grounds of futility. In the US it is advocated that patients should be informed of decisions made on the grounds of futility.[28] In the UK this is not thought to be necessary.[4,23]

- occasionally it may be justified to make DNR decisions on competent patients because of poor quality of life, without obtaining consent. This is permissible when it is thought that discussing CPR with patients is likely to be detrimental to their general wellbeing.[14]

- if a competent patient indicates that he or she does not wish to discuss CPR

Discussing DNR decisions with patients' relatives and friends

Discussions with relatives have a different focus from discussions with patients. Doctors should consider their responsibility for maintaining confidentiality, particularly since some patients may not want their relatives involved in decisions.[5,8]

Competent patients

Permission should be sought from the patient to speak to relatives.[14]

A DNR decision is considered on "poor quality of life" grounds and the patient has indicated that he or she does not wish to discuss this, or it is thought to be detrimental to his or her wellbeing. Discussions should aim to determine the patient's views of his or her quality of life and life prolonging treatment.

Incompetent patients

The doctor decides about treatment in the best interest of the patient. If DNR is being considered on the basis of "poor quality of life" then the doctor will usually want to get a better idea of what the patient would have wanted from relatives or friends. The doctor should also try and determine if there is an Advance Directive (living will), which now has legal force in Britain (see below).

It is usually a matter of good practice to inform relatives about an incompetent patient's progress and this is often straightforward.[24] There may be occasions, however, where different family members have different views or there have been family disputes. In these circumstances the obligation remains to make a decision in the best interest of the patient and only to share information with those whom the patient would have wanted it shared with.

What to tell patients about CPR

For consent to be valid it must be fully informed. Patients should be told the likely outcome of the procedure and about any major complications.

CPR is usually unsuccessful although many doctors, including those with recent experience of it, overestimate its success.[32] Survival depends on patient selection, but about 10% to 20% of those having CPR survive to leave hospital; most of these are still alive one year later, and long term neurological deficits are relatively uncommon, although 1-2% survive in a persistent vegetative state.[11,29] Survival is lowest for those on general wards with chronic illness. Selected elderly patients can do as well as selected younger ones, and old age should not be used as the basis for making DNR decisions, but elderly inpatients with chronic illness probably have a less than 5% survival to discharge.[19]

Doctors should try and estimate the success rate for the individual, mentioning the possibility of survival with neurological damage. They should ensure that patients know that if they have a cardiorespiratory arrest and do not have CPR then they will almost certainly die.[24]

Ideally, experienced clinicians (usually consultants)[1,14] should undertake such discussions. They should initially try to determine how much, if at all, the patient wishes to get involved in decisions about life prolonging treatments. If it is clear that the patient does not wish to discuss the issue then the doctor should seek permission to share information with a relative or friend.[14] Doctors should also discuss the implications of DNR decisions for other life prolonging treatments.

Written information given to patients on admission to hospital could include a description of CPR and a statement about the hospital's resuscitation policy.[14] Patients should then be given the opportunity to discuss this further with medical staff if they wish or to indicate if they would find this distressing.

Future developments

The courts have recently confirmed that Advance Directives have some legal force in Britain, and doctors should consider the possibility of there being a living will when making decisions for incompetent patients.[33,34] The BMA has produced a code of practice[34] to help health professionals understand the current situation in respect of living wills. Recent recommendations from the Law Commission, if accepted,[24] will clarify the position on Advance Directives and will provide a facility for patients to nominate another person to make healthcare decisions on their behalf in the event of incompetence.

The Commission proposes that the term "Advance Refusal" may be appropriate since it will usually refer to treatment that the

123

patient does not want in certain circumstances; if a patient requests treatment in advance which is not indicated clinically then there is still no obligation to use it.

The Commission's other proposal is that the Power of Attorney legislation should be modified so that a proxy could make decisions on behalf of an incompetent adult on health matters, not just on financial ones. The proxy would be obliged to make decisions in the best interest of the patient within a framework of safeguards. There is a separate proposal that, where there is no advance refusal or nominated proxy, doctors should consult widely about what is in the best interest of the patient. It is suggested that there should be consultation with "other people whom it would be appropriate and practicable to consult about the person's... best interest". This is probably what many doctors do already and the Commission avoids nominating specific relatives who should be consulted recognising that decisions have to be made "in a world of divided families".

Conclusions

In the future patients and their relatives will probably want more involvement in resuscitation decisions, so doctors need a sound knowledge of the ethical and legal basis on which decisions are made. A policy of discussing CPR with all patients on admission is impractical, unnecessary and may not be what patients want. It is possible that many elderly patients might be excluded from discussions because of incompetence or because CPR is futile. Discussions will inevitably be time consuming, should involve senior clinicians, and should be detailed enough to include individual information about the likely outcome of CPR. Written information given to all patients on admission could give details of the hospital's CPR policy and how patients can arrange to have further discussions about it. Doctors will be helped by the development and refinement of Advance Directives, but should be aware that some forms of Advance Directive already have legal force.

1   Decisions relating to cardiopulmonary resuscitation—a statement from the BMA and RCN in association with the Resuscitation Council (UK). London: British Medical Association, 1993.

2   Williams R. The Do Not Resuscitate decision: guidelines for policy in the adult. *J Roy Coll Phys Lon* 1993,27:139-46.

3   Florin D. "Do Not Resuscitate" orders: the need for a policy. *J Roy Coll Phys Lon* 1993;27:135-8.

4   Florin D. Decisions about cardiopulmonary resuscitation. *BMJ* 1994;**308**:1653-4.

5   Mead GE, Turnbill CJ. Cardiopulmonary resuscitation in the elderly: patient's and relatives views. *J Med Ethics* 1995;**21**:39-44.

6   Gunasekera NPR, Tiller DJ, Clements LTS. Elderly patients' views on cardiopulmonary resuscitation. *Age Ageing* 1986;**15**:364-8.

7   Hill M, MacQuillan G, Heath DA, Forsyth M. Cardiopulmonary resuscitation; who makes the decision? *BMJ* 1994;**308**:1677.

8   Morgan R, King D, Prajapati C, Rowe J. Views of elderly patients and their relatives on cardiopulmonary resuscitation. *BMJ* 1994;**308**:1677-8.

9   Potter JM, Stewart D, Duncan G. Living wills: would sick people change their minds? *Postgrad Med J* 1994;**70**:818-20.

10 Liddle J, Gilleard C, Neil A. The views of elderly patients and their relatives on cardiopulmonary resuscitation. *J Roy Col Phys Lon* 1994;**28**:228-9.

11 Saunders J. Who's for CPR? *J Roy Col Phys Lon* 1992;**26**:254-7.

12 Bayliss RIS. Thou shalt not strive officiously. *BMJ* 1982;**285**:1373-5.

13 Calman K. Health Service Commissioner - Annual report for 1990-91 Resuscitation policy. PL/CMO(91)22. 26.12.92.

14 Doyal L, Wilsher D. Withholding cardiopulmonary resuscitation: proposals for formal guidelines. *BMJ* 1993;**306**:1593-6.

15 Bellos A. Patient "can be allowed to die". The Guardian 1996. April 27th.

16 Bruce-Jones P, Bowker LK, Cooney V, Roberts H. Cardiopulmonary resuscitation: what do patients want? *J Med Ethics* 1996;**22**:154-9.

17 Wall JA, Palmer RN. Resuscitation and patients' views. *BMJ* 1994; **309**: 1442-3 (letter).

18 Diem SJ, Lantos JD, Tulsky JA. Cardiopulmonary resuscitation on television; miracles and misinformation. *NEJM* 1996;**334 (24)**:1578-82.

19 Murphy DJ, Burrows D, Santilli S, *et al.* The influence of the probability of survival on patients' preferences regarding cardiopulmonary resuscitation. *NEJM* 1994;**330**:545-9.

20 Robertson GS. Resuscitation and senility; a study of patients' opinions. *J Med Ethics* 1993;**19**:104-7.

21 Heller A, Potter J, Sturgess I, Owen A, McCormack P. Resuscitation and patients' views; questioning may be misunderstood by some patients. *BMJ* 1994;**309**:408.

22 Gillon R. *Philosophical Medical Ethics.* Chichester: John Wiley, 1986.

23 Doyal L, Wilsher D. Withholding and withdrawing life sustaining treatment from elderly people; towards formal guidelines. *BMJ* 1994;**308**:1689-92.

24 Mental Incapacity. Law Commission (No 231). London: HMSO, 1995.

25 *The living will: consent to treatment at the end of life.* Age Concern Institute of Gerontology and Centre of Medical Law and Ethics. London: Edward Arnold, 1988.

26 Rights and Responsibilities of Doctors. London: BMA, 1992.

27 Aarons EJ, Beeching NJ. Survey of "Do Not Resuscitate" Orders in a District General Hospital. *BMJ* 1991;**304**:1504-6.

28 Tomlinson T, Brody H. Ethics and communication in Do Not Resuscitate decisions. *NEJM* 1988;**318**:43-6.

29 Blackhall LJ. Must we always use CPR? *NEJM* 1987;**317**:1281-4.

30 Wagg A, Kinirons M, Stewart K. Cardiopulmonary resuscitation: doctors and nurses expect too much. *J Roy Col Phys Lon* 1995;**29**:20-4.

31 Weijer C, Elliott J. Pulling the plug on futility. *BMJ* 1995;**310**:683-4.

32 Waisel DB, Truog RD. The cardiopulmonary resuscitation not indicated order: futility revisited. *Ann Intern Med* 1995;**122**:304-8.

33 Doyal L. Advance Directives. *BMJ* 1995;**310**:612-3.

34 Advance statements about medical treatment. Report of the British Medical Association. London: 1995.

12 Sudden death of a family member

JONATHAN MARROW

Patients in the United Kingdom who die suddenly are very likely to be taken to the nearest hospital accident and emergency department. Death may follow collapse or the deceased may be found apparently lifeless. Severe injuries may prove fatal (box 12.1).

Major advances have been made in developing sound procedures for resuscitation of those suffering sudden cardiac arrest and also for the efficient management of victims of major life threatening trauma. Training in these procedures is seen as a high priority for doctors and nurses in many disciplines as well as for paramedic ambulance staff and other emergency personnel.

Application of the principles of Advanced Cardiac Life Support (ACLS), Advanced Trauma Life Support (ATLS) and Advanced Paediatric Life Support (APLS) should reduce the number of people who are brought in dead to accident and emergency departments and increase the proportion of those arriving in a critical condition who leave the department alive. It is absolutely right that we strive to develop and maintain our practical life saving skills in these areas but there is another aspect of the care of the critically ill or injured which deserves more attention.

When a death has to be confirmed in the accident and emergency department, there will normally be relatives or friends to be found and informed. Death has usually come quite unexpectedly, making the task of sharing the news all the more difficult. The suddenly bereaved effectively become our patients, every bit as deserving of our care as the person who has died.

> **Box 12.1 Some important causes of sudden death in adults***
>
> - myocardial infarction
> - road traffic accident
> - deliberate self poisoning
> - cerebrovascular accident
> - accidental carbon monoxide poisoning
> - alcohol intoxication and inhalation of vomit
> - asphyxia due to smoke inhalation
> - pulmonary embolism.
>
> *not in order of frequency

Apart from fulfilling a clear duty, providing proper care for the recently bereaved has an important role in reducing future psychiatric morbidity.[1] There have been many local initiatives regarding this aspect of care in the accident and emergency department.[2,3,4,5] The Department of Health has issued useful, but rather general, guidelines in its document *People who die in hospital.*[6] The recent excellent publication, *Bereavement care in A&E departments,*[7] is greatly to be welcomed but the care of the suddenly bereaved has still in general not been given the high national profile allotted to improving our efforts at resuscitation.[8]

We are naturally reluctant to admit the possibility (in some situations, the high probability) that resuscitation will fail. Also, formal teaching of the practical skills of life support seems much more straightforward than that of communication in the tragic crisis. Learning what to say and how to say it is one component. Learning to listen, and to be aware of non-verbal communication, is just as important and for many it is even harder to learn.[9]

Sharing feelings beyond your personal experience

Most health care professionals will have to make use of their imagination to begin to grasp the feelings of the person who has suffered sudden personal loss. The ability mentally to place yourself in the position of another individual is hard to teach, but can greatly improve the care given to a person who has to hear news of sudden bereavement.

There must, for example, inevitably be a great gulf in life experience separating any working doctor or nurse and a newly widowed 85 year old whose spouse has just died after 60 years of

127

marriage. The only way this can be bridged is by imagination, together with a habit of study of other individuals. The opportunity for such study is one of the great privileges of medical and nursing practice. It demands continuing awareness of the feelings of patients in all sorts of clinical situations.

While the task of initial care for those suddenly bereaved very often falls on staff of the accident and emergency department in the United Kingdom today, it is by no means their monopoly. The skills involved need to be as widespread as those of the various forms of life support.

Where to talk with bereaved relatives

Every accident and emergency department should have a room which can be set aside for the exclusive use of the family of a seriously ill patient, or one who has recently died.[2,4,5] The room should be comfortably furnished and decorated in a domestic rather than a clinical way. It needs to be sufficiently close to the resuscitation area for the family not to feel they are being separated excessively from their loved one. It should be secluded from public gaze. The room may sometimes be used for interviewing other relatives or for other occasional uses, but it must be available and tidy for immediate use at any time. It is not appropriate for a registrar's office or a staff rest room to double as a room for bereaved relatives.

Box 12.2 Accommodation in the accident and emergency department

Room for distressed relatives
- private
- quiet
- in or near accident and emergency department
- telephone
- access to washroom and toilet.

Room for viewing body
- private
- "in use" indicator panel on door
- suitable decor, non-denominational
- close to accident and emergency department, without obstructing care of new patients
- accessible without long delay
- relatives need to be able to touch and hold, not just view through window.

Relatives must have news, even when it is bad

Relatives often arrive when colleagues are still trying to resuscitate a patient who has suddenly collapsed, or been brought by ambulance from the scene of an accident. They deserve information and should be kept informed as quickly as possible. The uncertainty of waiting for news of someone you love is in many ways more painful than knowing what is happening, even if the news is bad. The desperate anxiety which families experience makes time seem to stop moving, so that minutes drag like long hours. The hectic activity of the resuscitation has the reverse effect on the time perception of staff involved.

Before the interview to break bad news

The need to tell the relatives what is happening is pressing, but there is still time to pause and check you have the essential facts. Make sure you know the patient's name, and be aware if there is any doubt about his or her identity. Have some detail of the patient's build and clothing in your mind to help make sure. Check that you have the latest facts about the patient's condition. Try to find out to whom you are going to speak.

Box 12.3 Before you talk to bereaved relatives

- ensure privacy
- seek non-clinical, comfortable environment
- try to make time, so that you are not rushed or disturbed
- make sure you will not leave the bereaved person alone after the interview
- is support available?
  - nurse or other health care professional
  - relatives or friends
  - appropriate religious support
- check your facts
  - identification of deceased. Is there any doubt about who has died?
  - identification of relatives. Who are you going to talk to?
  - what has the relative already been told?
  - will you be able to answer likely questions about patient?
- check your appearance
  - take off blood-stained gloves, gown, etc.

Case history 12.1

- a rural setting in Africa, night time
- a British wife is at home with her small child
- she is eight months pregnant
- her African husband dies in a car accident.

- young mother is woken by a friend driving round the house for half an hour before calling (he cannot think what to say)
- news is broken by a friend of her late husband, but he is too shaken to give clear information
- the widow has no opportunity to see her late husband
- there is no system of death certification.

- wise relatives in Africa enable the widow and her daughter to return to her own family (contrary to local custom)
- she is allowed to fly home, though heavily pregnant (contrary to airline regulations).

- supportive extended family in UK helps the young widow cope with conflict of grief for her husband, versus joy for the new baby
- lack of death certificate means a long delay before widowed mothers' allowance is payable
- the widow is too busy not to cope, but always has uncertainty about extent of her husband's injuries, because she did not see him herself.

The bereaved relative as your patient

Peoples' reactions vary a lot. You are unlikely to have met the family before but suddenly you are going to shake their world. You will leave impressions they are unlikely to forget. Up to now, your skills will mainly have been focused on your patient who is dying, or has died. You need consciously to turn your attention onto the person you are going to meet, regarding them now as a patient in need of your care in their own right. Some departments now follow the practice of registering the bereaved relative as a patient, which can be a helpful reminder of this need.

A nurse to support the bereaved family

It is a good idea to try to take someone with you, preferably an experienced nurse. Someone needs to stay with people who have just received bad news about a person close to them, to listen to their further questions, to comfort and support them. This is particularly important when the bereaved person is alone, of course. The ideal is that one person, usually an experienced nurse, can be freed of other duties in order to act as the named nurse, allocated to stay with the bereaved family, supporting them and, where necessary acting as an advocate for their interests.

Honesty when the outlook is poor

My title refers to breaking news only of sudden death, but often there is a preliminary stage, when the patient is clearly desperately ill and news has to be given to a relative who has come to the hospital. Honesty has to be the key. If you do not know what is wrong, it is best to say so, explaining that every effort is being made to find out the diagnosis. It is important to make sure that the family do realise when the outlook is very poor. They will very much want to be told, after all, that things are not as bad as they at first seemed. It is sometimes necessary gently but clearly to repeat statements in this situation.

Giving relatives access to the dead or dying

It is very important to be with a close family member, able to see them and hold them, when they are ill or injured. Families who have not been allowed to be with someone who has died suddenly can feel as if they have let their loved one down by not being there before he or she died.[10]

Box 12.4 Seeing the person who has died

- opinions differ about relatives being present during resuscitation (widely accepted with children)
- opportunity should always be offered to see body as soon as possible after death
- should be encouraged but never forced
- clear explanations of visible injuries or therapeutic interventions will be needed
- allow relatives to touch and hold their loved one
- allow a lock of hair to be cut, if it is requested
- be ready to support bereaved relatives but also be ready to give them privacy with deceased (if legal situation allows)
- time with deceased should be as unrushed as possible
- polaroid photograph should be offered, and retained if not wanted at time

---

Some suggest that the best way for the close kin of a gravely ill patient to appreciate what is happening, and to realise how hard staff are striving to keep them going, is for the relative to be with them, even in the hospital resuscitation room.[11] There is a tradition among staff that relatives will be too upset by medical procedures during resuscitation (and may get in the way). There is also probably a self consciousness about carrying out emergency procedures with an "audience". From departments where it is routine practice, it seems that relatives in the resuscitation room do not cause as much stress for staff as might have been expected.

The implications of inviting relatives into the resuscitation area do need to be carefully thought through. Different groups of medical and nursing staff need to be consulted and careful arrangements made. It is already the usual practice in some hospitals to invite relatives to visit the resuscitation room while resuscitation is in progress. Some allow it occasionally. Not all relatives accept, and there should certainly be no coercion. The

---

Box 12.5 Special problems

- sudden death of children
  - sudden infant death
  - sudden death in accident
  - sudden death in apparently avoidable circumstances
- death by criminal violence
  - grief and anger
  - needs of police
  - media attention
- the bereaved person is also seriously hurt
  - they need to be awake enough to understand
  - must consult rest of family but do not delay breaking news too long
- communication difficulties
  - language
  - disability
  - bereaved children
- cultural factors
  - religious obligations
  - beliefs and traditions of grieving
- relative on telephone
  - locally
  - at long distance, overseas
- media enquiries to you and to the family

---

practice is particularly favoured in paediatric accident and emergency departments. The named nurse responsible for the family should stay with the relatives in the resuscitation room, ready to offer explanation and support and also to judge if it is time to return to the relatives' sitting room.

The interview

Importance of honesty

Being at the hospital, even for a short time, before the close relative has died, can seem to make adjustment to sudden bereavement a little easier, even in a sudden accident or illness. However, the process of grieving and acceptance of loss has to be truncated, in any case.

It used to be a common practice that the family would first be told that the patient was desperately ill, even when they were actually dead already. They would later be told that resuscitation had been to no avail. It was done with the best of motives, to try to ease the blow of sudden bereavement, but I would advocate a more

---

Box 12.6 With the bereaved relatives

- build a bridge
  - introduce yourself
  - put yourself on a level with them physically
- establish relative's current information
  - what happened before sudden illness or accident?
  - what do they know about the sudden illness/accident?
- be alert to verbal and non-verbal signs from relative
  - be ready to confirm direct question "Is he/she dead?"
- do not prolong the agony of not knowing
  - if there has been no direct question, be ready to give brief account of injury or illness and, with regret, explain that treatment has not been successful and that relative has died
- use clear language, expressed with sympathy, but usually avoiding euphemisms
- listen - be responsive to the relative's reaction
  - follow with a more detailed explanation
  - go on listening, do not plough on, stifling the relative's questions and reactions
  - many relatives now ask about organs for transplantation. Have initial answers and be ready to make prompt enquiries

---

honest policy. Untruths are revealed, for example, when a family member is on the hospital staff or when a relative realises that death was actually confirmed before the first telephone call summoning the family to hospital was received. It is so important that the bereaved family can carry on, adjusting sadly to their loss but confident that they have been in touch with developments throughout. An open, honest approach will maintain trust, even if at first it seems unkind.

The interview as a consultation

Superficially, the interview to break the news of sudden death may appear simply to be a one way process—a meeting where the doctor or nurse gives information to family members. I suggest that it should better be approached as a consultation with a new patient. You do have information which has to be given, but you will do the job much better if you are prepared for an exchange. You need to be alert for signs from the relative or family group. Early on you will gain information about their current understanding and attitudes, which may guide you how best to explain what has happened. Later, when they know of their loss, the reactions and questions of the bereaved family will indicate what further facts you need to tell them, or find out, and also what further support may be needed.

Box 12.7 Some common reactions
- disbelief
  - "Are you sure he/she is dead?"
  - "Could there have been some mistake?" (of identification)
- guilt
  - "If only I had made him go to the Dr"
  - "I should have stopped him driving when he was tired"
- anger
  - against the deceased
  - against previous medical care
  - against you
  - against God
- unusual reactions (occasionally needing psychiatric help)
  - resolute denial, even after seeing the body
  - violent anger
  - disclosure of long-standing family strife, suspicions, accusation

---

> ## Case history 12.2
>
> - a young mother has been fatally injured
> - a heavy girder fell off a lorry and crashed into her family car
> - the dead woman was the front seat passenger
> - her husband, the car driver, was not physically injured.
>
> - "I know she is dead, doctor."
>
> - he tried to help the doctor who sat down to break the news
> - he had held his wife after the accident
> - he knew the extent of her injuries
>
> - the young husband was deeply distressed though calm on the surface
> - there were two young children
> - he kept asking if they would be taken into care
> - he needed to talk about breaking the news to his children
> - he needed reassurance that he and they could work out their own future lives
> - relatives came and were practical and supportive
>
> - in working out the care of his bereaved children, their father was able to start to come to terms with his own grief. The family stayed together.

You need to say who you are and establish with whom you are speaking. Try to put yourself on a level with your new patient, physically as well as in human terms. Sit with them, rather than standing over them. They may already have a very good idea what has happened. Try to sound out what they know about the sudden illness or accident but do not go on too long before sharing the bad news you have come to tell. Your manner needs to be appropriate to the situation. The way you choose to describe what has happened needs to be gauged according to the person you are talking to, their age and likely understanding of medical language, for example. There are many euphemisms surrounding the end of life; most are used to avoid the discomfort of recognising the speaker's own mortality. They may be open to misunderstanding and are usually better avoided.

Reactions to bad news

People's reactions in the situation of sudden bereavement vary enormously. Tears, questions, anger, doubt, and guilt are just some

135

of the facets. Some people will be so calm and quiet that you are unsure if you have expressed yourself clearly. Others will quietly thank you and offer sympathetic support to you, conscious of how difficult the task of breaking bad news must be.

The work of doctors and nurses is often seen to require a degree of detachment from violent emotions. Too close involvement can, indeed, sometimes make it difficult to reach rational decisions about patient care. This does not mean that they do not have feelings, of course. Recognising your own distress when a patient has died shortly after admission to hospital, for example, can make you better able at least to appreciate the level of the grief of those more personally involved.

Box 12.8 Information the bereaved family will need

- procedures about clothing and possessions
- explanation of Coroner's procedures and registration
- written details about formalities necessary after a death (registration, etc)
- written details of contact they can make for more explanation (with department)
- facts about transplantation, if requested
- possibilities of medical use for bodies, again, if requested.

The place of physical contact

Human touch is an important part of communication, particularly in the way we show sympathy or shared emotion. Touching a hand or arm or putting an arm round the shoulders of a person in distress can express our shared feelings far more effectively than words. Each person must find his or her own comfortable level. There is no prescribed correct way. You should not feel that you have to get closer than you feel is comfortable or natural.

Sensitivity to the needs of religious groups

Religion and culture play a large part in our attitude and reaction to death. We need to be ready to help with requests relating to religious needs, particularly as many groups feel that it is their duty to carry out rituals correctly at the time of death.[12] It is a unique moment for the one who has died and the family will feel they have failed him or her for ever if the chance is missed. There should be hospital chaplains for the main denominations but it is helpful to keep lists of contact names and telephone numbers for ministers of religion in the area of your hospital. A list of interpreters available in the hospital and in the community is also very useful.

Helping with legal formalities

There are procedural details which families need to know. There are usually legal obligations relating to sudden death (such as reporting the death to the Coroner in England and Wales, or the Procurator Fiscal in Scotland). Registration of death needs to be explained. A postmortem examination may be legally required, which will need great tact if there are cultural or religious objections.[13] If possible have the facts available. Be ready quickly to find out a detail, if you do not have the information straightaway. The shock of acute grief makes it very difficult to retain information so well laid out leaflets are very useful. Translations should be available where there is linguistic diversity, too.

Box 12.9 Headings for a policy on bereavement care in an accident and emergency department

- training of staff involved in the care of the bereaved
- responsibility for breaking bad news
- support for bereaved families in department (named nurse)
- maintenance of room for distressed relatives and viewing room
- maintenance of information for staff and for the bereaved (telephone numbers and leaflets, for example)
- registration of bereaved relatives as patients
- protocol about presence of relatives during resuscitation
- protocol on viewing of the deceased by relatives
- list of agencies to be informed when a death has occurred in department
- procedures about the property of deceased relatives (including clothing)
- support offered from accident and emergency department after the initial bereavement (contact name and phone number, home visits, visits to specialist clinic where relevant)
- support of staff involved in care of the bereaved.

Questions about transplantation

Questions about transplantation are often raised. When death has already occurred the possibilities for organ donation are usually limited to use of the corneas, but these alone are very valuable and you should know how to arrange for them to be used if it is possible in your area. Legal formalities (for example with the Coroner in England and Wales) need to have been agreed beforehand. Knowledge that at least some good has come out of a sudden death can bring great comfort, particularly if the family know it would have been the wish of the person who has died.

Clothing and other property

Great distress can be caused by lack of thought about clothing or valuable property after a sudden death. The family will need explanation when clothing has had to be cut off and warning about possible soiling. Clothing may have been retained by police officers if there is a possibility of violence, and the family need to be told this. It can be a kindness to have the clothes quickly washed through but some relatives feel that washing their loved one's clothes for the last time is at least one thing they can do in a situation where they feel very helpless. Wherever possible, the decision should be theirs.

Bereavement and children

The death of a child is a specially hard loss and caring for the distressed family when a baby has been found to have died suddenly is particularly gruelling.[14] This is discussed in chapter 3.

Helping children who have suffered bereavement is another very

---

Box 12.10 Some important causes of sudden death in children★

- sudden infant death syndrome (SIDS)
- meningococcal septicaemia
- road traffic accident
- home accident
- bronchial asthma
- epilepsy complications.

★not in order of frequency

Case history 12.3

- A young man, recently separated from his wife, attended an accident and emergency department with back pain
- After careful assessment, a simple strain was diagnosed and he was allowed home to rest
- He collapsed on his way home and died soon after being brought back to the hospital
- Medical and nursing staff were profoundly shocked as there had been no indication that he had been in danger when he first left hospital.

- The patient had not wanted staff to contact his wife when he first attended. He had not even given her address, because of the separation
- Staff did contact the young man's father in law by telephone while resuscitation was still going on
- He was to contact his daughter and she would come to hospital

- The young woman phoned first. By now her husband had died. The sister who spoke to her was herself shaken by the unexpected death. This was obvious in her speech. She felt that she had to tell the caller honestly what had happened. She had no idea of the cause of death.

- The death was reported to the Coroner and a postmortem showed a massive pulmonary embolus. The source was not found.
- The young widow spoke to the coroner's officer on the next day but did not come to hospital. The Coroner accepted that the death had been due to natural causes
- The widow did not know where to turn for more information.

- A week later, at the request of the widow's GP, the consultant arranged to meet the widow and she was grateful for a full explanation of what was known about what had happened
- She accepted that the death was a completely unexpected tragedy.

Lessons
- no policy can provide for every eventuality
- the emotions, even of experienced professionals, give themselves away, on the telephone as well as face to face
- when staff feel awkward, and perhaps guilty, about a patient's death, an early meeting with relatives is particularly important
- especially when a postmortem has shown an unusual cause for sudden death, hospital medical staff must take the initiative in seeking to talk to the family about it.

> ## Box 12.11 Afterwards
>
> - bereaved family may need help with transport home
> - may need overnight accommodation at hospital until morning
> - may need long talk with staff member best known to them (often a nurse who has sat with them while they waited for more news)
> - family doctor should be informed by quickest possible route
> - bereaved family may want to ask for more information later
> - should have opportunity to talk again with hospital staff, preferably named doctor or nurse, if they request it.

difficult area. They may attend with adult relatives but may, occasionally, be the only uninjured survivor in some family tragedy. There is not room in this short article to discuss the issues in any detail. Essentially, children need understandable information and support. They need to be told what has happened. After suitable explanation they should be allowed to see the body of the dead parent, if they wish to. They need to be allowed to react in their own way. Care for them by other relatives or if necessary by official agencies needs to be worked out. The help of the paediatric ward may be enlisted for a bereaved young child, for example pending the arrival of relatives from a distance.

Care for the bereaved after returning home

Some departments have arrangements for some after care following sudden bereavement. A dial-in telephone number to ring and a named nurse or doctor to ask for can be helpful when queries arise after the family have left hospital. Hospital staff will not wish to take over the role of the family doctor, but an opportunity to discuss the postmortem report with a doctor who was involved in the patient's care at hospital can be helpful. Uncertainties linger terribly, making adjustment to loss especially difficult and prolonged.

Care for staff working with sudden bereavement

Finally, the needs of hospital staff involved in the care of the suddenly bereaved need to be considered.[14,15] They need every help in carrying out this very difficult and gruelling task. They need training and preparation for it and they deserve support to help them with the stress it can induce. While often this can be on an informal basis, there needs to be a support structure for staff which allows access to more formal counselling when required. Staff need to be able to seek this help without feeling that it is an admission of failure.

I am particularly indebted to Dr Ed Glucksman and his colleagues on the working group from the British Association for Accident and Emergency Medicine and the Royal College of Nursing for their most valuable publication "Bereavement care in A&E departments." This work includes extensive discussion of the issues briefly covered in this chapter, together with an extensive list of useful addresses and a full bibliography.

1　Lundin T. Long term outcome of bereavement. *Brit J Psych* 1984;**45**:424-8.
2　Yates DW, Ellison G, McGuiness S. Care of the suddenly bereaved. *BMJ* 1990;**301**:29-31.
3　Tachakra SS, Beckett MW. Dealing with death in the accident and emergency department. *Brit J A and E Med* 1986;**1**:10-11.
4　Burgess K. Supporting bereaved relatives in A&E. *Nursing Standard* 1992;**6**:19:36-9.
5　McLauchlan CAJ. Handling distressed relatives and breaking bad news. *BMJ* 1990;**301**:1145-9.
6　Department of Health. *NHS Guidelines - patients who die in hospital HSG(92)*. London: Department of Health, 1992.
7　Working Group of British Association for Accident and Emergency Medicine and Royal College of Nursing. *Bereavement care in A&E departments*. London: Royal College of Nursing, 1995.
8　Cooke MW, Cooke HM, Glucksman EE. Management of sudden bereavement in the accident and emergency department. *BMJ* 1992;**304**:1207-9.
9　McManus IC, Vincent CA, Thom S, Kidd J. Teaching communication skills to clinical students. *BMJ* 1990;**301**:1145-7.
10　Renner S. I desperately needed to see my son. *BMJ* 1991;**302**:30-56.
11　Doyle C. Family participation during resuscitation - an option. *Ann Emerg Med* 1985;**10**:7-9.
12　Black J. Broaden your mind about death and bereavement in certain ethnic groups in Britain. *BMJ* 1987;**295**:536-8.
13　Sherwood SJ, Start RD. Asking relatives for permission for a post-mortem examination. *Postgrad Med Journal* 1995;**71**:269-72.
14　Brown P. Saying goodbye. *Nursing Times* 1993;**89**:26-9.
15　National Association for Staff Support. *A charter for staff support (for staff in Health Care Services)*. London: NASS, 1992.

13 Asking relatives for permission for a postmortem examination

SIMON J SHERWOOD, ROGER D START

There is increasing concern regarding the current world-wide decline in clinical or hospital postmortem rates.[1] The reason for this concern is that the postmortem is still of benefit to both medical practice and to society. The decline is believed to be due to a number of complex factors.[1] Clinicians, particularly junior clinicians, are usually responsible for approaching relatives for their permission[2-8] although in some cases specially trained decedent affairs staff may undertake this task.[9] These individuals therefore have a key role in determining hospital postmortem rates. This is particularly true in those countries which are now changing from a system whereby patients or relatives had to opt out of clinical postmortem to a system in which relatives' consent must be obtained.

A major factor in the decline in hospital postmortem rates is that fewer requests are being made.[3] This may be due to a number of reasons including a fear of confronting the relatives,[1] personal discomfort,[10,11] an inability to explain adequately the value of the postmortem,[12] a belief that relatives are becoming more reluctant to give permission,[5] or a desire not to upset the relatives.[11,13]

The outcome of an autopsy request is highly dependent on the manner in which it is made.[14] Thus, the process would be easier for all concerned if those involved in making the requests had received appropriate training and if the requesting procedures were well established.[9]

Training in requesting permission for a hospital postmortem

A large number of clinicians appear to have never received any formal training or advice in how to approach relatives for permission for a postmortem.[2,8,10,15,16] Most clinicians learn through personal experience or by accompanying senior colleagues who have had no training themselves.[10,16] Initial experiences could have long term effects on clinicians' motivation and expectations regarding future requests, particularly if these experiences are negative. This is one reason why preparation via the provision of relevant training is important.

Many junior clinicians feel that there is a need for training in how to request postmortems.[5,15,17] Support for this proposal has come from a wide range of clinical and non-clinical sources.[3,12,13,18,19,20,21] It has been suggested that most basic skills required for medical practice should be acquired during the pre-registration year when supervisors have a responsibility to ensure that adequate training is provided[22].

Content of training

The content and format of communication skills training should ideally be based upon a thorough assessment of training needs and the defined aims and objectives of the training programme.[23] Those requiring training might include medical students, clinicians, and/or relative support staff. The General Medical Council recommends that "Doctors must be good listeners... and they must be able to provide advice and explanations that are comprehensible."[22] More specifically, one of the objectives of the training programme might be to enable the appropriate individuals to request permission for hospital postmortems in a sensitive and understanding manner which allows the relatives to make informed decisions and minimises the risk of causing additional distress. Certain knowledge, skills and abilities might be relevant to training designed to reach this objective.

Individuals should be able to anticipate and cope with the reactions and concerns of relatives at the time of a bereavement. They should also be aware of possible religious and cultural sensitivities relating to death, funeral arrangements, and postmortem examinations.[12,13,19,21,24,25] An appreciation of the administrative procedures, and the roles and responsibilities of those involved with the death of a patient in hospital is also important. Agencies within the hospital include clinicians, and nursing, relative support, administrative and mortuary staff together with the pathologists. Agencies outside the hospital include the coroner's office (or equivalent authority), the office of the registrar of births, deaths and marriages, funeral directors, as well as the relatives of the deceased. There should also be an appreciation of the role of other agencies such as pastoral support, voluntary and charitable organisations.

Box 13.1 Deaths reportable to the coroner

A death should be referred to the coroner if the medical practitioner cannot readily certify death as being due to natural causes within the terms of regulation 51 of the Registration of Births, Deaths and Marriages Regulations 1968. Some of the circumstances in which a death might be reported include those in which:

- there are any suspicious circumstances or a history of violence
- the death may be linked to an accident (whenever it occurred)
- the deceased was receiving a war pension or industrial disability pension (unless the death can be shown to be wholly unconnected)
- the death may be due to industrial disease or may be related in any way to the deceased's employment
- the death is linked with an abortion
- the death occurred during an operation, or before full recovery from the effects of anaesthesia, or was in any way related to the anaesthesia
- the death may be related to a medical procedure or treatment
- the death may be due to a lack of medical care
- allegations of medical mismanagement have been made
- the actions of the deceased may have contributed to his or her own death
- the death occurred during or shortly after detention in police or prison custody
- the deceased was not seen by a doctor within the 14 days prior to death

(adapted from an article by Start et al [26])

Before making a postmortem request, clinicians must recognise the circumstances in which they should report a patient death (see box 13.1) to the coroner (or equivalent authority).[26] In some cases the circumstances in which death should be reported may be desired local practice rather than statutory requirements. It is important that clinicians who go to work in other countries familiarise themselves with the local guidelines—for example, in the US the circumstances may vary from state to state.[27] Individuals should also be able to explain the difference between medicolegal and hospital postmortems and the circumstances in which they are carried out. It seems that many of the public are unaware of this difference and a request might cause anxiety because of a belief that the cause of death is not known or that there are suspicious circumstances surrounding the death of their

---

Box 13.2 Reasons for refusal of a postmortem

- concerns about disfigurement and further suffering
- lack of information concerning the reasons for the postmortem
- not seeing the point of it
- dislike the thought of it
- too upset to consider it
- perceived stress of giving permission
- objections from other family members
- respect for the deceased and their wishes
- lack of information concerning the reasons for the postmortem
- religious/cultural objections (eg, from Jews, Muslims, Christian Scientists, Zoroastrians, the Afro-Caribbean community and Rastafarians)
- concern over possible interference with funeral arrangements
- a desire to conclude matters as soon as possible
- concerns about the cost

Box 13.3 Reasons for consent for a postmortem

- desire to help others
- to establish precise cause of death
- confirmation of diagnosis
- assist medical science and research
- wishes of the deceased
- wishes of other family members
- peace of mind
- reassurance about care provided
- recommendation of medical staff
- organ donation

---

relative. Clinicians should also be aware of the legal issues surrounding postmortems, such as who has the authority to give consent for such an examination.[19]

Clinicians should also be able to explain the cause of death using terminology which will be easily understood by the relatives. An understanding of relatives' misconceptions regarding postmortem examinations and the reasons why relatives refuse or give permission is a necessary basis for making effective requests and may alleviate possible fears and anxieties on the part of the relatives (see case histories 13.1-13.3).[12,18,24,28,29,30,31,32,33] The most frequent reasons given by relatives for refusing or giving permission for a postmortem are given in boxes 13.5 and 13.6.[13,17,19,24,25,34,35,36,37,38] Although clinicians are probably aware of most of these reasons, the influence of a lack of understanding of the need for a postmortem and fears over interference with funeral arrangements may not be fully appreciated.

In making a request the individual responsible should be able to explain the specific reasons why requests are made, and the benefits and continuing importance that postmortems can have for the medical profession, relatives and for society.[12,13,15,19,21,24,32,33,36,39] Relatives can find the request insensitive and may be distressed

---

Case history 13.1—A relative's concerns
Possible mutilation and disfigurement

A son is concerned that a postmortem examination would result in his mother's body being cut up and practised upon by medical students leading to disfigurement. In particular, he does not like the idea of any interference with her head as he wishes to have an open casket at the funeral service.

Reassurances

- the postmortem examination is similar to a surgical operation and is carried out by medically qualified pathologists
- the outward appearance of the deceased would not be altered in any way and no external marks would be visible
- if preferred, the next of kin could opt for a limited postmortem examination (which could specify avoidance of the head) or a needle core biopsy. (These options are only available in non-medicolegal cases where consent is required from the next of kin.)

Case history 13.2—A relative's concerns

Possible interference with funeral arrangements

A wife wishes to have her husband's body transferred to his home town for burial. As there are relatives travelling in from overseas to attend the funeral, she needs to make the necessary arrangements as soon as possible. She is worried that a postmortem examination might cause a delay.

Reassurances

- postmortem examinations take only a short time to perform and would not impede the release of the body to the funeral director
- in urgent cases postmortem examinations can be expedited or relatives can opt for a limited examination
- the mortuary staff can liaise with the funeral director in order to ensure that the body can be released and transferred in a timely fashion
- again, these options are only applicable to non-medicolegal autopsies.

because of a lack of warning, poor timing, or a failure to explain the reasons for the requests.[36,40] Medical students are often not informed of the value and utility of the postmortem examination and this will clearly influence their subsequent perceptions of its value.[1,10,21] Although some clinicians still appear to recognise the importance of postmortems, there is evidence to suggest that they are not aware of the full extent and nature of the information that they can provide (see boxes 13.4 to 13.6).[15,25]

The request should be made in a manner that does not put

Box 13.4 The benefits of the postmortem

For the medical profession
- establishes a precise cause of death
- improves the accuracy of epidemiological statistics
- gives feedback on the accuracy of clinical diagnosis
- gives information on the effects of (new) drugs, treatments, surgical procedures, and disease processes
- aids undergraduate/postgraduate medical education
- aids medical audit and risk management
- enables research and advancement of knowledge

Box 13.5 The benefits of the postmortem

For the relatives

- knowledge of precise cause of death
- confirmation of diagnosis
- reassurance and peace of mind
- alleviation of guilt through reassurance that death was inevitable and that all appropriate care was taken
- assistance in the advancement of medical knowledge
- an opportunity to help others
- assistance with the grieving process
- identification of possible hereditary conditions and diseases and infectious diseases
- assistance with insurance and compensation claims

Box 13.6 The benefits of the postmortem

For the society in general

- improved accuracy of epidemiological statistics
- organ and tissue donation
- identification and monitoring of occupational and environmental health hazards
- identification and monitoring of infectious diseases and epidemics
- increase in medical knowledge

---

pressure on relatives, who should be given time to consider and discuss their decision (perhaps with others) if they so wish.[19,21] The clinician should have an understanding of the nature of postmortems and the possible alternatives to a full examination (eg, limited postmortem, needle core biopsy, or laparo/endoscopic examination[33,41,42,43,44]) together with the practicalities involved with the arrangement of the examination and the dissemination of the results.[19,33] This would enable them to deal with any questions raised by relatives; for example, relatives are often left unsure as to whether they will be informed of the results and how they will be communicated.[38]

A suitable training programme must promote the necessary knowledge, skills, and abilities as well as a positive attitude towards the issue of requests for postmortems. For example, clinicians should be encouraged to take responsibility for ensuring that relatives who give consent receive the results of the examination as

---

Case history 13.3—A relative's concerns

Lack of understanding of the justification for a postmortem examination

A sister does not understand what possible benefits could be gained from a postmortem examination if the cause of her elderly brother's death is already known.

Reassurances

- the postmortem may provide useful information which was not available when the patient was alive
- postmortem examinations can be beneficial, not just to the medical profession, but also to the relatives and society in general, eg, through the demonstration of hereditary or infectious diseases
- the medical profession can gain vital feedback concerning the accuracy of clinical diagnosis and effects of treatment
- the results may assist relatives with the grieving process. It may be a comfort to know more about the cause of death and that all appropriate care was given.

---

soon as possible, and are also given an opportunity to discuss them with a clinician or a general practitioner.[3,12,32,45,46] Postmortem results are often delayed or may never reach the relatives at all.[3,36,40]

Ideally, formal training in requesting permission for postmortems should be part of a comprehensive programme designed to provide a range of communication skills appropriate to dealing with death and dying.[12,47] There appears to be growing acceptance of the need for formal communication skills training within this type of educational context which is directly relevant to clinical practice.[48,49]

Benefits of training in how to request permission for a hospital postmortem

The provision of relevant training could increase clinicians' motivation to request a postmortem by increasing their perceptions of its value and by increasing their confidence in their ability to approach relatives. Such training might also make them feel more comfortable with the task and increase their expectations of gaining permission.[50] Improvements in the quality of the requests made could lead to increases in hospital postmortem rates due to greater success rates in gaining permission.[31] Improvements could also reduce the likelihood of causing additional distress to relatives, which is an obvious concern of clinicians, and could lead to a better and more accurate understanding of the nature and importance of the postmortem by the general public.

How is communication skills training being provided?

The most commonly used teaching methods for communication skills training in the UK medical schools are tutorials, video feedback, role playing and lectures.[48,51,52] Self-teaching workshops, and group discussion appear to be less frequently used. It is difficult to draw conclusions about the relative frequency of the use of real and simulated patients because of differences in the level of data collected in these surveys. Teaching methods are clearly an important issue since the effectiveness of training will be dependent on these methods as well as on the complexity of the required skills.[53] There are currently insufficient data to assess the relative effectiveness of different teaching methods.[48]

Clinicians appear to prefer more active teaching techniques such as small group seminars and tutorials, group discussion, and the use of demonstration videos, video feedback sessions and role play. More passive teaching methods including written guidelines and lectures are considered to be less desirable.[10] Most UK medical schools seem to be striving to move away from lectures towards more small group learning.[22]

When is communication skills training provided?

More than a third of all communication skills training in British medical schools[48] appears to be provided during the first clinical year. There is growing support for the introduction of integrated communication skills training which would begin in the undergraduate curriculum and continue into postgraduate and continuing medical education.[48,49,54,55] Other suggestions have been that it would be difficult to provide training at the undergraduate level and that this might best be provided at the beginning of the pre-registration year.[22,57] Some clinicians consider the most

150

desirable time for such training to be between the beginning of the final undergraduate year and the end of the pre-registration year.[10]

The ideal communication skills training programme may be one which provides training at appropriate times during the undergraduate medical education (for example, postmortem requests could be introduced during the teaching of pathology) and then reinforces key skills of direct relevance to specific areas of clinical practice in the pre-registration year, in postgraduate and in continuing medical education.

1 Hill RB, Anderson RE. *The autopsy - medical practice and public policy.* Boston: Butterworths, 1988.

2 Chana J, Rhys-Maitland R, Hon P, Scott P, Thomas C, Hopkins A. Who asks permission for an autopsy? *JR Coll Physicians Lond* 1990;**24**:185-8.

3 McPhee SJ, Bottles K, Lo B, Saika G, Crommie D. To redeem them from death: reactions of family members to autopsy. *Am J Med* 1986;**80**:665-71.

4 Harris A, Ismail I, Dilly S, Maxwell JD. Physicians' attitudes to the autopsy. *JR Coll Physicians Lond* 1993;**27**:116-8.

5 Wilkes MS, Link RN, Jacobs TA, Fortin AH, Felix JC. Attitudes of house officers toward the autopsy. *J Gen Intern Med* 1990;**5**:122-5.

6 Kesler RW, Maxa V, Saulsbury FT. Evaluation of physicians' requests for autopsies. *J Med Educ* 1983;**58**:153-5.

7 Katz JL, Gardner R. Request for autopsy consent. *NY State J Med* 1973;**1**:2591-6.

8 Inglis FG, McMurdo ME. Post-mortem rates and junior doctors in Tayside—three years after the Joint Working Party report. *Health Bulletin* 1995;**53**:379-85.

9 Haque AK, Cowan WT, Smith JH. The decedent affairs office: a unique centralized service. *JAMA* 1991;**266**:1397-9.

10 Sherwood SJ. Motivation to request permission for hospital autopsies: the predictive utility of clinicians' strength of self-efficacy, outcome expectations, and outcome values. MSc Dissertation. Sheffield, England: University of Sheffield, 1993.

11 Birdi KS. A comparison of the theory of planned behaviour and the theory of reasoned action in the context of requesting hospital autopsies. (MSc dissertation). Sheffield, England: University of Sheffield, 1992.

12 Charlton R. Autopsy and medical education: a review. *JR Soc Med* 1994;**87**:232-6.

13 Report of the Joint Working Party of the Royal College of Pathologists, the Royal College of Physicians of London and the Royal College of Surgeons of England. *The autopsy and audit.* London: Royal College of Pathologists, 1991.

14 McGoogan E. The autopsy and clinical diagnosis. *JR Coll Physicians Lond* 1984;**18**:240-3.

15 Hinchliffe SA, Godfrey HW, Hind CRK. Attitudes of junior staff to requesting permission for autopsy. *Postgrad Med J* 1994;**70**:292-4.

16 Katz JL, Gardner R. The intern's dilemma: the request for autopsy consent. *Psychiatry Med* 1972;**3**:197-203.

17 Stolman CJ, Castello F, Yorio M, Mautone S. Attitudes of pediatricians and pediatric residents toward obtaining permission for autopsy. *Arch Pediatr Adolesc Med* 1994;**148**:843-7.

18 Brown HG. Perceptions of the autopsy: views from the lay public and program proposals. *Hum Pathol* 1990;**21**:154-8.

19 Connell CM, Avey H, Holmes SB. Attitudes about autopsy: implications for educational interventions. *Gerontologist* 1994;34:665-73.

20 Inglis FG, McMurdo ME. The death of the postmortem. *Scott Med J* 1995;40:131-2.

21 The Scottish Office Home and Health Department Scottish Health Service Advisory Council. *Autopsy Services in Scotland: A Report by the National Advisory Committee for Scientific Services.* Edinburgh: The Scottish Office Home and Health Department, 1994.

22 The General Medical Council Education Committee. *Tomorrow's doctors: recommendations on undergraduate medical education.* London: The General Medical Council, 1993.

23 Patrick J. *Training research and practice.* London: Academic Press, 1992.

24 Green J, Green M. *Dealing with death: practices and procedures.* London: Chapman Hall, 1992.

25 Lazda EJ, Brown DC. An audit of autopsy rates in an inner London general hospital. *JR Soc Med* 1994;87:658-60.

26 Start RD, Delargy-Aziz Y, Dorries CP, Silcocks PB, Cotton DWK. Clinicians and the coronial system: ability of clinicians to recognise reportable deaths. *BMJ* 1993;306:1038-41.

27 Schmidt S. Consent for autopsies. *JAMA* 1983; 250: 1161-4.

28 Sanner MA. In perspective of the declining autopsy rate. *Arch Pathol Lab Med* 1994;118:878-83.

29 Sanner MA. Medical students' attitudes toward autopsy: How does experience with autopsies influence opinion? *Arch Pathol Lab Med* 1995;119:851-8.

30 Start RD, Saul CA, Cotton DWK, Mathers NJ, Underwood JCE. Public perceptions of necropsy. *J Clin Pathol* 1995;48:497-500.

31 Clayton SA, Sivak SL. Improving the autopsy rate at a university hospital. *Am J Med* 1992; 92: 423-8.

32 Webster JR, Derman D, Kopin J, Glassroth J, Patterson R. Obtaining permission for an autopsy: its importance for patients and physicians. *Am J Med* 1989;86:325-6.

33 Berger LR. Requesting the autopsy: a pediatric perspective. *Clin Pediatr* 1978;17:445-52.

34 Geller SA. Religious attitudes and the autopsy. *Arch Pathol Lab Med* 1984;108:494-6.

35 Gatrad AR. Muslim customs surrounding death, bereavement, postmortem examinations, and organ transplants. *BMJ* 1994;309:521-3.

36 Start RD, Sherwood SJ, Kent G, Angel CA. Audit study of next of kin's satisfaction with clinical necropsy service. *BMJ* 1996;312:1516.

37 Solomon SA, Adams KHR. Attitudes of relatives to autopsies of elderly patients. *Age and Ageing* 1993;22:205-8.

38 Kirkham N, Renshaw M. Next of kin satisfaction with the autopsy. *J Pathol* 1993;170:374A.

39 Start RD, Hector-Taylor MJ, Cotton DWK, Startup M, Parsons MA, Kennedy A. Factors which influence necropsy requests: a psychological approach. *J Clin Pathol* 1992;45:254-7.

40 Witter DM, Tolle DM, Mosley JR. A bereavement program: Good care, quality assurance, and risk management. *Hospital & Health Services Administration,* 1990;35:263-74.

41 Schneiderman H, Gruhn JG. How- and why- to request an autopsy. *Postgrad Med* 1985;77:153-64.

42 Foroudi F, Cheung K, Duflou J. A comparison of the needle biopsy post mortem with the conventional autopsy. *Pathol* 1995;27:79-82.

43   Avrahami R, Waternberg S, Daniels-Philips E, Kahana T, Hiss J. Endoscopic autopsy. *Am J Forensic Med Pathol* 1995;**16**:147-50.
44   Avrahami R, Waternberg S, Hiss Y, Deutsch AA. Laparoscopic vs conventional autopsy, *Arch Surg* 1995;**130**:407-9.
45   Whitty P, Parker C, Prieto-Ramos F, Al-Kharusi S. Communication of results of necropsies in North East Thames region. *BMJ* 1991;**303**:1244-6.
46   Hutchins GM. Practice guidelines for autopsy pathology. Autopsy reporting. Autopsy Committee of the College of American Pathologists. *Arch Pathol Lab Med* 1995;**119**:123-30.
47   Field D. Formal instruction in United Kingdom medical schools about death and dying. *Med Educ* 1984;**18**:429-34.
48   Whitehouse CR. The teaching of communication skills in United Kingdom medical schools. *Med Educ* 1991;**25**:311-8.
49   Consensus statement from the Workshop on the Teaching and Assessment of Communication Skills in Canadian Medical Schools. *Can Med Assoc J* 1992;**147**:1149-50.
50   Cottreau C, McIntyre I, Favara BE. Professional attitudes toward the autopsy: a survey of clinicians and pathologists. *Am J Clin Pathol* 1989;**92**:673-6.
51   Frederikson L, Bull P. An appraisal of the current status of communication skills training in British medical schools. *Soc Sci Med* 1992;**34**:515-22.
52   McManus IC, Vincent CA, Thom S, Kidd J. Teaching communication skills to clinical students. *BMJ* 1993;**306**:1322-7.
53   Maguire P. Can communication skills be taught? *Br J Hosp Med* 1990;**43**:215-6.
54   Parle J, Wall D, Holder R, Temple J. Senior registrars' communication skills: attitudes to and need for training. *Br J Hosp Med* 1995; **53**: 257-60.
55   Heavey A. Learning to talk with patients. *Br J Hosp Med* 1988;**39**:433-9.
56   Jolly BC, MacDonald MM. Education for practice: the role of practical experience in undergraduate and general clinical training. *Med Educ* 1989;**23**:189-95.

Index

Page numbers printed in **bold** type refer to figures; those in *italic* to tables or boxed material

INDEX